Clinical Decision Making
for the
Physical Therapist Assistant

Clinical Decision Making
for the
Physical Therapist Assistant

Steven B. Skinner, PT, MS, EdD
Kingsborough Community College
City University of New York
Brooklyn, New York

Christina McVey, PT, MA
Kingsborough Community College
City University of New York
Brooklyn, New York

JONES AND BARTLETT PUBLISHERS
Sudbury, Massachusetts
BOSTON   TORONTO   LONDON   SINGAPORE

World Headquarters

Jones and Bartlett Publishers
40 Tall Pine Drive
Sudbury, MA 01776
978-443-5000
info@jbpub.com
www.jbpub.com

Jones and Bartlett Publishers
Canada
6339 Ormindale Way
Mississauga, Ontario L5V 1J2
Canada

Jones and Bartlett Publishers
International
Barb House, Barb Mews
London W6 7PA
United Kingdom

Jones and Bartlett's books and products are available through most bookstores and online booksellers. To contact Jones and Bartlett Publishers directly, call 800-832-0034, fax 978-443-8000, or visit our website, www.jbpub.com.

Substantial discounts on bulk quantities of Jones and Bartlett's publications are available to corporations, professional associations, and other qualified organizations. For details and specific discount information, contact the special sales department at Jones and Bartlett via the above contact information or send an email to specialsales@jbpub.com.

Production Credits

Publisher: David Cella
Associate Editor: Maro Gartside
Production Manager: Julie Bolduc
Associate Production Editor: Jessica Steele Newfell
Marketing Manager: Grace Richards
Manufacturing and Inventory Control Supervisor: Amy Bacus

Cover Design: Scott Moden
Cover Image: © Taewoon Lee/ShutterStock, Inc.
Interior Design: Shawn Girsberger
Composition: Glyph International
Printing and Binding: Cenveo
Cover Printing: Cenveo

Library of Congress Cataloging-in-Publication Data

Skinner, Steven B.
  Clinical decision making for the physical therapist assistant / Steven B.
Skinner, Christina McVey.
    p. ; cm.
  Includes bibliographical references and index.
  ISBN 978-0-7637-7125-6
  1. Physical therapy assistants. 2. Physical therapy assistants--Decision
making. I. McVey, Christina. II. Title.
  [DNLM: 1. Physical Therapy Modalities. 2. Allied Health Personnel. 3.
Clinical Medicine--methods. 4. Decision Making. 5. Decision Support
Techniques. 6. Orthopedic Procedures--methods. WB 460 S628c 2011]
  RM701.S65 2011
  615.8'2023--dc22

                                                                2009052346

6048

Printed in the United States of America
14 13 12 11 10   10 9 8 7 6 5 4 3 2 1

Dedication

This text is dedicated to the memory of Emma Jean Beverly, a dedicated wife, loving mother, doting grandmother, and great mother-in-law.

—SBS

To my greatest fan, Bob. Thank you for all your encouragement and support. All my love.

—Christina

To my Emily. Always reach for the stars and enjoy what you do. Love always.

—Mommy

Contents

Preface   xiii

About the Authors   xv

Chapter 1: Introduction to Decision Making   1

Understanding Pre-Established Goals   4

Attendance to the Rehabilitation Environment   4

    Interdisciplinary Team   4

    Rehabilitation Setting   5

    Accessing Available Resources   5

Understanding Patient/Family Needs   5

Utilization and Assessment of Objective Measures   6

Possession of Sound Clinical Knowledge and Expertise   7

The Range of Clinical Decisions   8

Limits on Clinical Decisions   9

Chapter 2: Clinical Decision Making in Communications   11

Goals of Treatment   12

Attendance to the Rehabilitation Environment   14

Altered Patient Status or Unexpected Physiological Responses   16

Patient Communication   16

References   18

What Do YOU Think?   19

**Chapter 3: Clinical Decision Making in Ethical
Provision of Physical Therapy Services**   21

Common Ethical Conflicts   23

References   25

What Do YOU Think?   26

Chapter 4: Clinical Decision Making in Gait Training   **29**

Goals of Gait Training   29

Attendance to the Rehabilitation Environment   30

Understanding Patient/Family Needs   31

Utilization and Assessment of Objective Measures   32

Progressive Ambulation Training with Assistive Devices   33

Possession of Sound Clinical Knowledge and Expertise   34

Limits on Clinical Decisions   37

References   37

What Do YOU Think?   38

Chapter 5: Clinical Decision Making in Administering Thermal Modalities   **41**

Goals of Treatment   41

Attendance to the Rehabilitation Environment   43

Understanding Patient Needs   44

Utilization and Assessment of Objective Measures   45

Possession of Sound Clinical Knowledge and Expertise   46

Limits on Clinical Decisions   48

References   48

What Do YOU Think?   49

Chapter 6: Clinical Decision Making in Administering Electrical Stimulation   **53**

Goals of Electrical Stimulation   54

Attendance to the Rehabilitation Environment   54

Understanding Patient/Family Needs   55

Utilization and Assessment of Objective Measures   55

Possession of Sound Clinical Knowledge and Expertise   55

Electrical Stimulation for Pain Management   56

Electrical Stimulation to Facilitate Muscle Contraction   58

Limits on Clinical Decisions   59

References   59

What Do YOU Think?   60

Chapter 7: Clinical Decision Making in Managing Neurological (CNS) Conditions   **65**

Goals of Treatment   65

Attendance to the Rehabilitation Environment   67

Understanding Patient/Family Needs   68

Utilization and Assessment of Objective Measures   69

Possession of Sound Clinical Knowledge and Expertise   71

Appreciation of the Relationship Between
the Sequelae and Function   74

Receptivity to Alternate or Blended Intervention
Strategies   76

Limits on Clinical Decisions   76

References   77

What Do YOU Think?   78

Chapter 8: Clinical Decision Making in Administering Therapeutic Exercise   **83**

Goals of Treatment   84

Attendance to the Rehabilitation Environment   85

Understanding Patient Needs   87

Utilization and Assessment of Objective Measures   88

Possession of Sound Clinical Knowledge and Expertise   89

Thinking Outside the Box   96

Limits on Clinical Decisions   98

References   99

What Do YOU Think?   100

Chapter 9: Clinical Decision Making in the Provision of Pediatric Physical Therapy Services   **105**

Goals of Treatment   106

Attendance to the Rehabilitation Environment   107

Understanding Patient Needs   110

Utilization and Assessment of Objective Measures   112

Possession of Sound Clinical Knowledge and Expertise   114

Limits on Clinical Decisions 116
References 116
What Do YOU Think? 117

Chapter 10: Clinical Decision Making in the Provision of Geriatric Physical Therapy Services **123**
Goals of Treatment 124
Attendance to the Environment 125
Understanding Patient Needs 127
Utilization and Assessment of Objective Measures 128
Possession of Sound Clinical Knowledge and Expertise 129
Limits on Clinical Decisions 132
References 133
What Do YOU Think? 134

Chapter 11: Clinical Decision Making in Prosthetic and Orthotic Training **141**
Goals of Treatment 141
Attendance to Environment 143
Understanding Patient Needs 144
Utilization and Assessment of Objective Measures 146
Possession of Sound Clinical Knowledge and Expertise 147
Limits on Clinical Decisions 148
References 148
What Do YOU Think? 149

Chapter 12: Clinical Decision Making in Managing Patients with Complex Acute Medical Conditions **155**
Treatment Goals 156
Attendance to the Environment 157
Utilization and Assessment of Objective Measures 159
Limits on Clinical Decisions 164
References 164
What Do YOU Think? 165

**Chapter 13: Clinical Decision Making
in Clinical Management** **169**

ORBIT 169

    Organize, Relate, and Bracket 170

    Integrate 171

    Treat 171

Application of the ORBIT Model 171

    Organize, Relate, and Bracket 173

    Integrate 174

    Treat 174

Conclusion 175

Index **177**

Preface

I t is difficult to count the number of clinical decisions physical therapist assistants (PTAs) make on a daily basis. Each clinical decision impacts the effectiveness of the physical therapy treatment and ultimately the patient's response to that treatment. Although physical therapists evaluate patients, design treatment plans, and may carry out most of the therapeutic plan, PTAs are expected to make decisions based on and within the scope of the plan of care entrusted to them. PTAs may make the following clinical decisions: resistive exercise dosage, determining the amount of assistance a patient needs during ambulation, or deciding the most effective way to communicate with a patient. Regardless of how prescriptive the treatment plan, in order to implement effective therapeutic activities PTAs are constantly called upon to use their knowledge while considering available resources and the goals of treatment.

The previous paragraph is demonstrative of the impetus for the writing of this text. As instructors of physical therapist assistants, the authors have painstakingly designed a curriculum with the goal of developing competent physical therapist assistants. They have observed students develop sound technical skills yet struggle with coupling technical prowess with true clinical decision making. When observing students carrying out simulated treatment plans, they have observed students face difficulty with queries such as: "Why did you choose that activity first?" "Why did you decide to start straight leg raises with 5 pounds?" "Why did you choose ambulation distance as the best indicator of progress?"

Even during clinical internships—though generally scoring high marks—students continue to struggle a bit with clinical decision making. Clearly, as clinicians mature and garner experience, their skills in this area improve—processes that seem to require conscious thought become more automatic. It is hoped that this text will jump-start the clinical decision-making process. Hopefully, this text will facilitate the notion of sound clinical decision making, starting in the first PTA foundation courses right through to the more advanced work.

Clinical Decision Making for the Physical Therapist Assistant is designed to not only make students aware of the clinical decisions that must be made but also to guide them on how to make those decisions. This book may be used at any stage of PTA education. Once the student completes a specific topic or skill in a particular course, the student may then read the corresponding chapter within this text. This book may also be used at the end of the formal educational program when students are expected to be able to pull all information together regarding patient treatments.

At the end of most chapters, the student is given the opportunity to answer critical-thinking questions. Additionally, most chapters contain treatment activities, where students can read an evaluation, perform a treatment on a simulated patient, and answer questions related to decisions made during the treatment.

Though some basic didactic information related to the topics covered in this text is provided, it should be clearly understood that this text is not meant as a review of content provided in individual PTA education courses. The basic information that is presented is provided as a reminder of decision-making factors and should not be considered exhaustive. The authors hope that this text adds to an important aspect of PTA education and plays at least a small role in the continued development of competent PTAs.

About the Authors

Steven B. Skinner, PT, MS, EdD

Steven B. Skinner is a physical therapy educator and clinician with 28 years of professional experience. He earned his physical therapy credentials from the University of Pennsylvania and holds a master's degree in adapted physical education and a doctorate in healthcare education. Dr. Skinner has worked as a clinician and administrator in several major New York metropolitan healthcare facilities. He has also owned and operated a private practice. Dr. Skinner currently serves as the Director of the Physical Therapist Assistant program at Kingsborough Community College of the City University of New York.

Christina McVey, PT, MA

Christina McVey is a physical therapy educator and clinician with 19 years of professional experience. She earned her physical therapy credentials from Quinnipiac College and holds a master's degree in health administration. Ms. McVey continues to work as a clinician, specializing in pediatrics and early intervention as well as general adult care. She currently serves as an assistant professor and Coordinator of Clinical Education for the Physical Therapist Assistant program at Kingsborough Community College of the City University of New York.

Introduction to Decision Making

Physical therapy assistants, or PTAs, are not physical therapy technicians. The term technician *suggests someone who is expert in the technical aspects of a task. Technicians read and execute orders. They are trained to be aware of contraindications and threats to safety and to act accordingly. Technicians are not called upon to make significant clinical decisions. PTAs, however, have greater responsibilities.*

It is best to start this discussion by acknowledging that most of us are master decision makers. As our cognitive development proceeds, our decision-making capabilities improve. From deciding which toy to play with to what career to enter, from determining how to cross a busy street to choosing the most appropriate treatment modality, decision making is enhanced through cognitive maturation, experience, and learning. Amazingly, many of our more routine decisions appear to be made automatically, with seemingly little conscious thought or effort. In contrast, complex decisions require more deliberate thought. It is clear, however, that the process used for simple and routine decision making is no different from that used for more complex problems. This text will attempt to illuminate and operationalize decision-making processes that enhance clinical practice in physical therapy.

Let's examine how you probably made the decision to become a PTA. Someone may have advised you to consider entering the field. He or she likely made that decision by observing your behavior and personality and concluding that physical therapy was a good fit for you.

You may have sought opportunities to observe physical therapy and PTAs in action. You may have compared your personal goals and desired lifestyle with a PTA's earning potential and other career factors to determine whether physical therapy was indeed right for you. You probably had to decide whether you possessed the appropriate science aptitude and caring attitude to succeed. Before making the final decision, you probably sketched out a plan—written or mental—as to how you could feasibly complete PTA educational requirements. After considering these and other factors, you then made the decision to become a PTA. Although you may not have engaged in this process in a steplike fashion, at some point during your career decision-making process you probably considered the factors mentioned. Your decision was based on: (1) understanding and setting goals, (2) analyzing personal needs and desires, (3) assessing limitations and strengths, (4) observing the environment, and (5) synthesizing a plan of action (**Figure 1.1**). These same factors (with some minor modifications) must be considered in clinical decision making.

In physical therapy, clinical decision making is a systematic process by which clinicians gather information, make judgments, establish

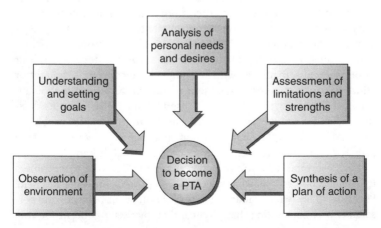

Figure 1.1 Decision-Making Factors

diagnoses, and synthesize plans of action to facilitate satisfactory progression toward established rehabilitation goals. Although they are not responsible for clinical decision making that leads to a diagnosis or the synthesis of a treatment plan, it is crucial that PTAs engage in effective clinical decision making with respect to appropriate clinical progression, assessment of intervention efficacy, and meeting patients' needs.

PTAs are often required to engage in significant clinical decision making. They must carry out treatment plans as designed by physical therapists. In carrying out those plans, PTAs must make important clinical decisions. These decisions may include the determination of the type of therapeutic exercise to administer, progression within therapeutic exercise and gait activities, selection and alteration of some physical agent parameters, and assessment-based modifications within the plan of care. When making clinical decisions, PTAs engage in a process that is dependent on their understanding of pre-established goals, attendance to the rehabilitation environment, an understanding of patient/family needs, assessment of objective measures, and the possession of sound clinical knowledge and expertise (**Figure 1.2**).

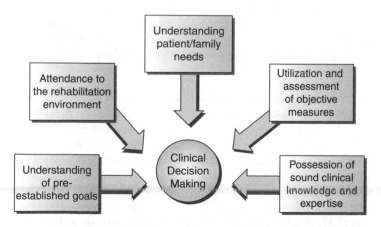

Figure 1.2 Clinical Decision-Making Factors

◖ Understanding Pre-Established Goals

Most physical therapy evaluations include the specification of treatment goals. Depending on the complexity of the patient's conditions, these goals may be more or less expansive in scope. For instance, the patient with a moderate shoulder adhesive capsulitis may emphasize joint range of motion and muscle strength, which are fairly moderate goals. However, treatment goals for a patient in a rehabilitation center with a diagnosis of cerebrovascular accident (CVA) will be much more extensive. The goals will most likely address movement/muscle coordination, gait, activities of daily living, joint range of motion, and so on.

It is crucial that PTAs understand the significance of the established goals. It is insufficient to simply catalog goals and treat them as merely a documentation exercise. Treatment goals can significantly affect clinical decision making. They may signal the relative aggressiveness of treatment, alter treatment emphasis, and/or influence intervention selection.

◖ Attendance to the Rehabilitation Environment

PTAs must be keenly aware of the overall rehabilitation environment when making clinical decisions. *Rehabilitation environment* refers to those external factors that impact the patient's rehabilitation. These factors include the interdisciplinary team, the rehabilitation setting, and expertise in identifying and accessing available resources.

Interdisciplinary Team

Depending on the case's complexity, the number of involved rehabilitation professionals may vary. PTAs' clinical decision making may be influenced by the types of additional rehabilitation services the patient is receiving. Physical therapy treatment must not take place in a vacuum. It is important that PTAs reach out to interdisciplinary team members and understand their rehabilitation goals and how they relate to the physical therapy goals. In in-patient rehabilitation settings, this typically takes place in formal and regular team conferences. However, it is equally important that regular interdisciplinary communication occurs in other, less formal settings.

Rehabilitation Setting

Clearly, the rehabilitation setting greatly influences the type and extent of clinical decisions PTAs may be called upon to make. Physical therapy services are provided in a wide variety of settings, including schools, specialty clinics, general private practices, acute care hospitals, nursing homes, subacute care facilities, and rehabilitation centers. In acute care settings, clinical decisions may be focused on moving patients to basic levels of function in preparation for the next level of care. In outpatient settings, clinical decisions may focus more on maximizing the patient's ability to perform activities of daily living. Regardless of the setting, PTAs are often called upon to make a vast array of clinical decisions to facilitate the accomplishment of treatment goals. Effective PTAs understand their provision of physical therapy care in the context of the rehabilitation setting and associated patient needs.

Accessing Available Resources

Clinical decision making is certainly influenced by the ability of PTAs to understand and access available clinical resources. Clinicians often become comfortable with doing things a certain way. They like to use a certain ultrasound machine. They avoid an unfamiliar electrical stimulation device. They perform therapeutic exercise in a stereotypical fashion. PTAs must ensure that their knowledge of available resources, rather than their comfort level with particular techniques and procedures, impacts clinical decision making.

PTAs must carefully survey the available clinical resources. For instance, they must know which ultrasound machines allow for frequency modifications, or which electrical stimulation units can provide interferential modes, or which exercise machines can provide variable resistance, and so on. A clear and complete knowledge of the available clinical resources surely enhances and influences the clinical decisions the clinician will make.

◀ Understanding Patient/Family Needs

It is important for PTAs to remember that effective rehabilitation requires the concerted efforts of both the clinician and the patient. This point must be communicated to the patient in very clear terms.

Modern Western society is very focused on instant gratification. If we are sick, we want a pill to get better. If we are a few pounds overweight, we want to shed them as quickly as possible with the least amount of work. Effective physical therapy treatment counters these societal desires. The clinician and patient must work together to achieve goals. Typically, patients must invest more time in achieving the designated rehabilitation goals than their therapists. To maximize rehabilitation, they must be compliant with home exercise programs, vigilant in maintaining appropriate postures, mindful of goals made in the clinic, and dedicated to applying successes to their activities of daily living.

Therefore, PTAs should strive to understand their patients' needs. PTAs should have some knowledge of their patients' premorbid conditions, family/work responsibilities, recreational status, and so on. Knowledge of these types of factors will influence clinical decisions such as rates of progression, types of home exercise programs, and modality use.

◀ Utilization and Assessment of Objective Measures

The knowledge of results certainly influences clinical decisions. How does a clinician know if treatment is effective? Pain scales, manual muscle testing, goniometry, isokinetic testing, circumferential measurement, and other assessments are crucial to efficacy assessment. PTAs use these types of assessments to attach an objective number or finding to their observations. Clearly, if a patient's initial shoulder abduction range of motion is 0 to 80 degrees and two weeks later it is 0 to 110 degrees, then there has been a measurable improvement. This change will significantly affect decision making. Such information may be used to alter how aggressive the stretching program should be, determine when to emphasize strengthening over stretching, or know when to consult with the physical therapist to alter the treatment plan.

It is easy for PTAs to fall into the habit of considering objective assessment as episodic rather than continuous occurrences. Assessment is not something that occurs only on a strict or prescribed schedule (e.g., interim and discharge summaries). Rather, assessment occurs continuously. Each treatment session should include at least some objective assessment, because assessment results guide the next step in the rehabilitation process. PTAs must strive to make assessment an integral part of all therapeutic activities.

◀ Possession of Sound Clinical Knowledge and Expertise

Clearly, all clinical decision making is undergirded by a sound understanding of the clinical, anatomical, physiological, and physical concepts applied in physical therapy. When involved in entry-level PTA education, students must not simply rely on rote memorization of facts. Students must strive to understand the presented material. They must work hard to apply the presented information to unfamiliar situations. They must strive to appreciate that although academic content is necessarily presented in separate classes, all coursework is intertwined and interconnected. They must be ever ready to apply presented material across the curriculum. Practicing PTAs must maintain their clinical and academic skills. They must take advantage of appropriate continuing education opportunities, participate in peer learning and investigation activities, and continuously strive to maintain and update their skills.

PTAs are not physical therapy technicians. The term *technician* suggests someone who is expert in the technical aspects of a task. Technicians read and execute orders. They are trained to be aware of contraindications and threats to safety and to act accordingly. Technicians are not called upon to make significant clinical decisions. PTAs have greater responsibilities. Their educational training provides them a more than cursory knowledge of physiological and clinical concepts. Additionally, PTA education includes a significant clinical component, providing students with opportunities to practice clinical decision making and hone physical therapy skills.

It is true that physical therapists synthesize treatment plans and goals. However, PTAs may have responsibility for carrying out all or part of the treatment plan. Within that responsibility resides a range of simple to complex decisions that may be made by PTAs. Such decisions can be effectively made only if the clinician indeed possesses sound clinical knowledge and expertise.

PTAs may be called upon to make a wide range of clinical decisions. The range of decisions exists on a continuum from simple to complex. Physical therapy treatment plans also exist on a continuum from more general to prescriptive. The type of plan provided may be dependent upon the type of facility, the patient's acuity, the relative level of PTA supervision, as well as clinician expertise and experience (PT/PTA). For example, let's assume a patient is referred to physical therapy following removal of a long leg cast for management of a distal femoral fracture. Following the initial evaluation, the physical therapist assigns the patient to a PTA. The physical therapy treatment plan includes *electrical stimulation to enhance quadriceps strength*. This part of the treatment plan is written in fairly general terms. Physical therapists assume that PTAs are capable of making the appropriate clinical decisions to carry out the treatment plan.

◀ The Range of Clinical Decisions

Such clinical decisions include the use of high-voltage or alternating current, as well as the determination of pulse frequency, duty cycle, electrode placement, and ramp/surge parameters (**Figure 1.3**). Clearly, the treatment plan may specify these parameters. However, in the

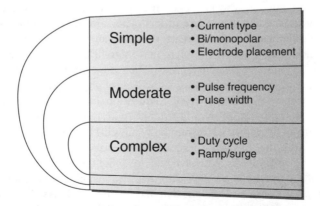

Figure 1.3 Potential Range of Clinical Decisions in Electrical Stimulation

absence of such specifications, to provide appropriate treatment PTAs must know what parameters they may alter without PT consent, when to obtain specific instructions from the physical therapist, and/or how to apply other clinical decision-making skills. The chapters in this text will examine various aspects of physical therapy treatment and identify the parameters and processes that facilitate sound PTA clinical decision making.

◀ Limits on Clinical Decisions

Just as PTAs may make a wide range of clinical decisions, they must be aware of the more prescriptive aspects of physical therapy care. Indeed, even routine physical therapy interventions may be strictly prescribed by physical therapists. More complex interventions such as iontophoresis, isokinetic strengthening, and postfracture gait training may be quite prescriptive. However, clinical decisions related to patient comfort and safety must still be made. Once strictly prescribed, PTAs must follow the treatment plan or consult the supervising physical therapist for changes to that plan.

Clinical Decision Making in Communications

2

Regrettably, in large or busy physical therapy settings, patients may be assigned to PTAs followed by minimal communication with the assigning PT. When this occurs, the rehabilitation process is compromised. PTAs work best as active members of the dual team rather than as quasi-independent clinicians performing interventions based solely on information gleaned from an initial evaluation, interim assessment, or previous progress note.

Though perhaps not as readily thought of as a clinical decision, PTAs must know and decide when they should formally communicate with the supervising PT. Effective PTAs extend the hands of PTs. They provide quality, prescribed physical therapy services that allow for the dual physical therapy team to impact a larger patient population than either the PT or PTA could serve alone. Effective PTAs must be comfortable in knowing what clinical decisions they may safely make and those that require PT consultation. PTAs who frequently query PTs about clinical issues that—based on their training—they should be able to handle may ultimately negatively impact the efficiency of the rehabilitation process. However, PTAs who make decisions that they are unqualified to make may negatively impact goal attainment and patient safety. Effective PTAs are expert in knowing when they must formally communicate with PTs. These statements do not negate the significance of the daily on-court chatter that should constantly occur between PT and PTA team members.

◀ Goals of Treatment

Effective PTAs carefully attend to the established goals of treatment. PTAs can sometimes become too focused on performing the technical aspects of the treatment. They become quite competent in providing simple and even some complex modalities, as well as guiding patients through therapeutic exercises and activities. However, the emphasis on goal attainment is sometimes diminished. Most PT written evaluations provide—in some form—treatment goals. In some instances, these goals are subdivided into long- and short-term goals. When the goals are subdivided in this way, it is easier for PTAs to remain focused on the goals. Regardless of whether the goals are subdivided into short- and long-term goals, PTAs must remain goal oriented. Nonachievement of goals or slow progression toward goal achievement certainly triggers the decision to communicate with the PT.

Effective PTAs realize that there is nothing magical about physical therapy. Ultrasound does not need to build up to some mystical physiological level before it is effective. The effects of resistive exercise do not appear in an instant, although they can be observed over a relatively short period of time. For the most part, successful pain management strategies produce near-immediate—though perhaps incremental—positive effects, or they are likely ineffective. Every therapeutic activity is associated with a therapeutic goal. PTAs must carefully catalog patients' progression toward goal achievement. When that progression slows or arrests, communication with the supervising PT is mandatory.

The tracking of progress is initially performed via written documentation. PTAs write progress notes on all patients under their care. The frequency of progress notes may differ based on the type of facility, patient acuity, and facility standards. Regardless of these variables, effective PTAs make the clinical decision to always write comprehensive progress notes. It may seem unusual to discuss notewriting in the context of clinical decision making. However, all clinicians can indeed make the decision to write more or less effective notes. PTAs often operate under significant time constraints. Patient caseloads are often large, necessitating occasionally *doubling* and sometimes *tripling* up patients in a 45- or 60-minute treatment session.

Many PTAs view notewriting as a necessary but laborious chore rather than a critical procedure in providing appropriate therapeutic techniques. Effective PTAs make the clinical decision to efficiently manage their time to maximize the potential for writing effective progress notes. The use of digital recorders, personal digital assistants (PDAs), and computer software may further facilitate effective notewriting. Sound documentation practices must be as highly prioritized as selecting and providing effective therapeutic interventions.

Note that written documentation can be considered the primary vehicle of communication between members of the multidisciplinary healthcare team. The adage "if it's not written, it's not done" often holds true. Effective documentation of provided treatment, patient response and progress, treatment plan, and so on is intricately linked to effective physical therapy and to third-party reimbursement. The latter association has led to the use of check-off, computerized, and other directed notewriting practices to ensure that clinicians document all critical information in an effort to reduce third-party payment denials.

Competent PTAs, whether using a more prescribed notewriting system or an open narrative style, such as the traditional SOAP (Subjective/Objective/Assessment/Plan) note, must make the clinical decision to always write complete and accurate notes. Clearly it is beyond the scope of this text to discuss the varied effective documentation strategies. Authors such as Wendy Bircher, Ginge Kettenbach, Eric Shamus, and Debra Stern have specifically addressed and outlined effective documentation practices for physical therapy clinicians. Sound notewriting reflects the basics of clinical decision making. Subjective data gleaned from the patient lead to objective parameters of treatment, including the selection of appropriate interventions and objective measurement tools. The results of the objective measures fuel the assessment of the efficacy of the chosen interventions and, in turn, influence treatment alterations and refinements to the plan of care (**Figure 2.1**).

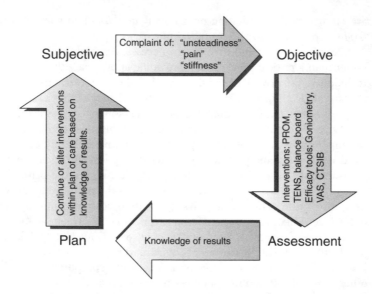

Figure 2.1 SOAP Note Reflection on Clinical Decision Making

◖ Attendance to the Rehabilitation Environment

Effective PTAs are sensitive to the status and changes in the rehabilitation environment and how they affect goal achievement. Critical changes in the rehabilitation environment must be reported immediately and discussed with the supervising PT (**Figure 2.2**).

Physical therapy is becoming more dependent on technology. Equipment malfunction may adversely affect goal achievement. PTAs must not hesitate in discussing critical equipment failures with the supervising PT. PTAs may believe that recently purchased equipment in other departments—a new fluidotherapy unit in occupational therapy, a multichannel biofeedback unit in speech therapy, or a new assessment regimen in vocational training—may be of benefit to one or more of their assigned patients.

Competent PTAs will initiate the discussion with the supervising PT and perhaps participate in interdisciplinary planning. Effective PTAs

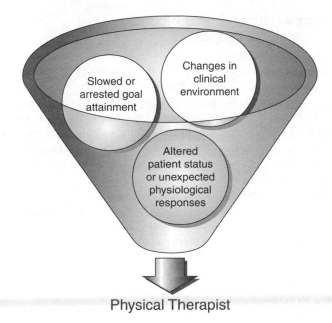

Figure 2.2 Factors Precipitating Communication

are lifelong learners. They read journal articles, scan professional periodicals for new techniques and procedures, and attend continuing education courses. When introduced to new concepts and ideas that may benefit assigned patients, effective PTAs formally discuss them with the supervising PT and, if feasible, participate in developing strategies to implement the new ideas into the plan of care.

PTAs appreciate the potential fluidity of the rehabilitation environment. They understand that there is no such thing as *routine treatment*. They remain vigilant in detecting factors that may influence goal attainment. Once detected, they must make the prudent clinical decision to communicate these factors to the supervising therapist.

◀ Altered Patient Status or Unexpected Physiological Responses

Superficial heating results in observable erythema. Progressive resistive exercise yields increased strength. Elevation and compression decreases edema. Cryotherapy limits inflammation. These reactions are grounded in basic physiological concepts and processes. They are the basis for the implementation of therapeutic modalities and procedures. There is little variation in the normal physiological responses to therapeutic procedures. When expected physiological responses do not materialize or do not precipitate expected results, effective PTAs readily make contact with the supervising PT.

Unfortunately, it is not unusual to review a physical therapy chart that documents multiple sessions of resistive exercise and with no significant change in strength or multiple episodes of modalities and stretching without appreciable changes in range of motion. In these cases, the chosen activities may not be appropriate or an underlying neuromuscular or medical condition may be limiting progress. As soon as the expected physiological response is not realized, PTAs must communicate formally with the supervising PT. Early detection and communication may prevent harm and lead to an early alteration in the plan of care or referral to other healthcare professionals for further evaluation.

Regrettably, in large or busy physical therapy settings, patients may be assigned to PTAs followed by minimal communication with the assigning PT. When this occurs, the rehabilitation process is compromised. PTAs work best as active members of the dual team rather than as quasi-independent clinicians performing interventions based solely on information gleaned from an initial evaluation, interim assessment, or previous progress note. Clearly, the supervising PT bears responsibility in ensuring appropriate communication. However, effective PTAs guard against this compromise by making the clinical decision to be proactive in communicating with the supervising PT.

◀ Patient Communication

Clinician–patient communication is often complex. It includes written, verbal, and nonverbal modalities. Effective PTAs recognize the barriers to patient communication and devise strategies that maximize effectiveness. Factors, including education level, central nervous system impairment, language difference, and hearing loss, may adversely affect how well PTAs communicate with their patients. **Table 2.1** presents common communication challenges and offers some effective coping strategies. PTAs understand that physical therapy effectiveness depends greatly on the ability to transmit information. The PTA must effectively discuss goals, explain therapy interventions, instruct therapeutic and self-management techniques, and communicate gains in functional terms.

The patient must effectively relate changes in symptoms, communicate personal needs and goals, and respond to clinical queries. Effective PTAs make the clinical decision to customize communication strategies for each patient. For instance, if a recently assigned patient with CVA is a retired mechanical engineer, the PTA may explain the use of a quad cane using terms such as *base of support* and *center of gravity*. Such terms might not be used with patients who do not have the same level of experience or education. The PTA makes the clinical decision to communicate with patients at the appropriate level to better achieve the therapeutic goals. Once again—as in all of physical therapy intervention—*one size does not fit all.*

Effective PTAs recognize the power of nonverbal communication. They make the clinical decision to maintain an upbeat and positive outward presentation when interacting with patients, regardless of whether less than optimal personal or clinical circumstances exist.

Table 2.1 Effective Communication Strategies

	Simple Instructions	Low Pitch	Nonverbal Cueing	Large Font	Simple Word Selection	Simple Gestures	Tactile Cues
Aphasia	X		X		X	X	
Cognitive impairment	X				X		
Hearing impairment		X	X				
Low level of education	X				X		
Sight impairment	X			X			X

Further, effective PTAs understand the importance of effective demonstration during patient instruction. The adage "a picture is worth a thousand words" may hold true in many patient encounters. The effective PTA makes the decision to be attuned to the patient's nonverbal behavior. Patients communicate their needs or responses to treatment in a variety of ways. Some may cry out when experiencing discomfort, whereas others may simply grit and bear it. In maximizing rehabilitation potential, PTAs must effectively discern each patient's communication style.

A significant amount of PTA interaction with patients is indeed instructional. PTAs may be considered "rehabilitation instructors." Gait training, therapeutic exercise administration, prevention measures, and other aspects of physical therapy all require PTAs to impart knowledge, assess mastery, and modify strategies—all of which are indeed teaching behaviors. PTAs must be mindful of the notion of the varying learning styles that patients possess. Although it is certainly beyond the scope of this text to fully explore motor learning and learning styles and preferences concepts, it is well known that individuals learn differently—attending to different aspects of the overall environment. Effective PTAs need not be learning experts. However, effective PTAs, when faced with unsatisfactory results, are able to alter their teaching behavior to facilitate the achievement of treatment goals.

Communication is complex. It requires sensitivity to differing styles and modalities as well as an understanding of what must be communicated. Effective physical therapy services cannot be provided if open lines of communication between clinician and patient, members of the interdisciplinary team, and other professionals are not established. Effective PTAs fashion communication strategies that support the attainment of physical therapy goals.

◀ References

Bircher, W. D. (2008). *Lukan's Documentation for Physical Therapist Assistants* (3rd ed.). Philadelphia: F.A. Davis.

Kettenbach, G. (2009). *Writing Patient/Client Notes: Ensuring Accuracy in Documentation* (4th ed.). Philadelphia: F. A. Davis.

Shamus, E., & Stern, D. (2004). *Effective Documentation for Physical Therapy Professionals.* New York: McGraw-Hill.

What Do YOU Think?

▶ **Scenario 1**

You are treating a patient with a history of Alzheimer's who has recently fractured her right leg, resulting in a long leg cast. What communication techniques can you use when teaching this patient to transfer out of bed and into a chair?

▶ **Scenario 2**

You are treating a patient who is blind and recovering from a right total hip replacement. What communication techniques can you use when teaching this patient about total hip replacement precautions?

▶ **Scenario 3**

You are treating a patient who is recovering from coronary bypass surgery with active range of motion (AROM) exercises, transfer, and ambulation training. The doctor asks you, as the PTA, how this patient is doing. What information would be important to convey to the doctor?

▶ **Scenario 4**

You are putting a patient with an open wound containing necrotic tissue and purulent discharge into a whirlpool tank. The wound does not have a pleasant look or odor. Discuss nonverbal communication that would *not* be appropriate in this scenario.

▶ **Scenario 5**

The physical therapist has assigned you a patient with a diagnosis of terminal cancer. The treatment plan includes bed mobility, transfer training, and pain management to make the patient as comfortable as possible. You enter the patient's room and the patient refuses physical therapy.

1. What would you do?
2. What needs to be communicated to the supervising physical therapist?

Clinical Decision Making in Ethical Provision of Physical Therapy Services

PTAs may find themselves in difficult ethical dilemmas not of their choosing. As an employee or subordinate rehabilitation partner, PTAs may be directed by PTs or others to perform in a less than ethical fashion. How do PTAs resist less than ethical directives? Surely the Nuremberg defense of "I was just following orders" is inadequate— both legally and ethically.

The ethical provision of physical therapy services is a top priority for all effective PTAs. Ethical performance of duties is emphasized in PTA education through role-playing in the laboratory and the review of ethical concepts in the classroom. The American Physical Therapy Association (APTA), through the Standards for Ethical Conduct for the Physical Therapist Assistant, provides guidelines for ethical conduct (**Figure 3.1**). Individual states, through specific legislation, regulate the overall practice of physical therapy and provide frameworks for the ethical performance of duties. Ethical performance of duties may be viewed as an either-or phenomenon. Ethical PTAs follow the guidelines of ethical practice in all situations. However, the minute their performance strays from the guidelines, they are considered to be practicing unethically and are subject to sanction.

Although this "black or white" viewpoint has merit, PTA conduct is greatly influenced by a variety of personal, organizational, and supervisory factors. These factors may cause PTAs to view ethical performance of duties as a continuum rather than in definitive terms (**Figure 3.2**). They may view the performance of duties in *degrees* of ethical conduct.

APTA Standards of Ethical Conduct for the Physical Therapist Assistant

PREAMBLE

This document of the American Physical Therapy Association sets forth standards for the ethical conduct of the physical therapist assistant. All physical therapist assistants are responsible for maintaining high standards of conduct while assisting physical therapists. The physical therapist assistant shall act in the best interest of the patient/client. These standards of conduct shall be binding on all physical therapist assistants.

STANDARD 1

A physical therapist assistant shall respect the rights and dignity of all individuals and shall provide compassionate care.

STANDARD 2

A physical therapist assistant shall act in a trustworthy manner towards patients/clients.

STANDARD 3

A physical therapist assistant shall provide selected physical therapy interventions only under the supervision and direction of a physical therapist.

STANDARD 4

A physical therapist assistant shall comply with laws and regulations governing physical therapy.

STANDARD 5

A physical therapist assistant shall achieve and maintain competence in the provision of selected physical therapy interventions.

STANDARD 6

A physical therapist assistant shall make judgments that are commensurate with their educational and legal qualifications as a physical therapist assistant.

STANDARD 7

A physical therapist assistant shall protect the public and the profession from unethical, incompetent, and illegal acts.

Figure 3.1 American Physical Therapy Association Standards of Ethical Conduct for Physical Therapist Assistants (Reprinted with permission from the American Physical Therapy Association. This material is copyrighted, and any further reproduction or distribution is prohibited.)

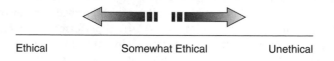

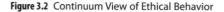

| Ethical | Somewhat Ethical | Unethical |

Figure 3.2 Continuum View of Ethical Behavior

For example, say that a PTA is instructed to not document or emphasize a patient's need for maximum assist sit-to-stand transfers because it will jeopardize the patient's transfer to a rehabilitation center. By not accurately documenting the patient's status, is the PTA performing in an unethical fashion? Have the PTA's actions actually harmed anyone, or have they helped the patient progress to the next level of care? If the PTA believes that the instructions are unethical, what are the consequences of refusal?

In this scenario, a PTA may recognize the unethical behavior but at the same time determine that it is just a little unethical and is required to move the patient to the next level or to ensure job security. Or, perhaps the PTA just does not want to rock the boat. Clearly, in an ideal world the decision to strictly follow ethical guidelines is easy. However, in the real world it is increasingly difficult. PTAs must make the clinical decision to provide physical therapy services in the most ethical fashion. This decision helps protect the integrity of the physical therapy profession as well ensure the rights and safety of the patient.

◀ Common Ethical Conflicts

The provision of physical therapy services is becoming increasingly complex. Private practices, hospitals, nursing homes, rehabilitation centers, and other facilities may experience financial stress and varying levels of administrative obligations to third-party payers and regulatory agencies. Sometimes responses to these stresses and obligations lead professionals to operate in a less than ethical fashion. Common ethical conflicts associated with these stresses and obligations include inappropriate documentation practices, the misuse of ancillary personnel, and inappropriate PTA supervision.

PTAs have an ethical and legal responsibility to accurately document physical therapy intervention. In some facilities, PTAs may be pressured to document intervention in less than accurate ways. For instance, if an inpatient refuses physical therapy and the assistant is unable to convince the patient to participate, the PTA may be instructed to write a note that suggests at least some services were provided (e.g., patient education, passive range of motion, etc.). If the minimum intervention duration is considered to be 30 minutes, the documentation of such services may suggest that the time requirement has been met—even if the PTA only spent 10 minutes with the patient. Once again, such a practice causes little actual harm. However, it does begin to chip away at ethical behavior, perhaps making it easier to behave in more unethical ways in the future. Here again, the PTA is following orders and may not necessarily view such documentation practices as unethical or may view them to be just a little unethical.

In an effort to manage costs, private practice owners may employ a variety of clinicians and nonskilled personnel, including athletic trainers, massage therapists, physical therapy aides, as well as physical therapist assistants. Sometimes the boundaries of duty and responsibility become blurred, and the ethical practice of physical therapy may be compromised. PTAs may find themselves in situations where they are required to write progress notes on treatment sessions that—at least in part—were carried out by inappropriately trained personnel. Even if not required to write such notes, continuing to work in a facility where unethical practices are the norm may lead to questioning a PTA's ethical values.

Individual state legislation regulates physical therapist supervision of PTAs. Standard 3 of the American Physical Therapy Association Standards of Ethical Conduct for Physical Therapist Assistants (Figure 3.1) specifically outlines the physical therapist supervisory role. However, PTAs may be placed in situations that compromise law and ethics. If the lone PT calls in sick and no coverage is available, should all patient appointments be cancelled, or should the PTA be allowed to treat his or her regular caseload? How should the PTA respond if instructed to treat patients that day?

PTAs may find themselves in difficult ethical dilemmas not of their choosing. As an employee or subordinate rehabilitation partner, PTAs may be directed by PTs or others to perform in a less than ethical fashion. How do PTAs resist less than ethical directives? Surely the Nuremberg defense of "I was just following orders" is inadequate—both legally and ethically.

When faced with ethical dilemmas, PTAs must carefully and systematically consider their actions. One approach to decision making is posing and answering several questions that may lead to prudent action (Kornblau & Starling, 2000). By posing questions, considering possibilities, brainstorming possible actions, and analyzing potential

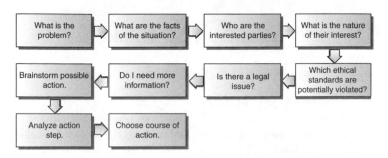

Figure 3.3 Clinical Decision-Making Process When Dealing with Ethical Dilemmas

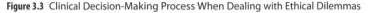

actions, PTAs may better be able to handle ethical issues as they arise. **Figure 3.3** represents this decision-making process.

Making the right ethical decisions may not always be easy. However, by maintaining high ethical standards, PTAs can play a laudable role in maintaining the integrity of the rehabilitation environment.

◀ References

Kornblau, B., & Starling, S. (2000). *Ethics in Rehabilitation: A Clinical Perspective.* Thorofare, NJ: Slack.

What Do YOU Think?

> ### Scenario 1 (Level I or II)

You are a PTA working in an outpatient physical therapy office. You arrive at work and find out that the only PT on staff has called in sick and you have been asked to see all the patients that day. (All new evaluations have been canceled.)

1. What would you do?
2. If you treated all the patients, what Standards of Ethical Conduct for the PTA would be violated?

> ### Scenario 2

A patient is being treated for knee pain with a hot pack and enters the clinic with complaints of shoulder pain. The patient wants you to treat her shoulder with a hot pack also.

1. What would you do?
2. If you gave the patient a hot pack to her shoulder, would you be in violation of state law?

> ### Scenario 3

You are working with another PTA and notice that he has asked the PT aide to give an ultrasound to one of his patients. The aide says yes and performs the ultrasound without any problems. What would you do?

> ### Scenario 4

You ask a patient how he is feeling. He says he is feeling pretty good. However, the patient tells you to make sure you explain just how poorly his knee is feeling and how poor his motion is on the progress note that is going to the workers' compensation board. (You think the patient could run out of the department if he had to.)

1. What would you do?
2. What would you tell the patient?

▶ **Scenario 5**

A patient is attracted to you, and you are attracted to the patient. The patient inquires about making your relationship personal as well as professional. What would you do?

Clinical Decision Making in Gait Training

4

Gait is complex. Neuromuscular, musculoskeletal, and psychological factors affect gait. PTAs must understand how these factors influence clinical decision making. Rather than simply identifying phases of gait, PTAs must understand the goals of those phases and how, through muscle contraction, momentum, and joint mechanics, human locomotion is possible.

PTAs spend a significant amount of time addressing gait issues. Gait training involves not only improving deviations, but also teaching safe and efficient ambulation with or without assistive devices. PTAs are required to make a wide range of clinical decisions during gait training. When making those decisions, PTAs must rely upon their observational skills, familiarity with assistive devices, and their knowledge of the objective parameters of gait. Once again, absent specific protocols, plans of care tend to be more general than specific. For instance, a patient with a diagnosis of CVA may present with a plan of care that reads, in part, "transfer and ambulation training" or "progressive ambulation training." PTAs are expected to possess the ability to appropriately progress a patient through a therapeutic gait program.

◖ Goals of Gait Training

PTAs must be very aware of the goals of prescribed gait training. The initial evaluation should clearly indicate the goals of gait training and answer the question "Why is the patient having difficulty

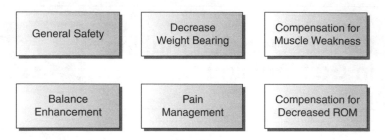

Figure 4.1 Major Therapeutic Goals for Gait Training

ambulating?" Cues within the initial evaluation guide the gait training program. These cues include diagnosis, mental status, weight-bearing status, range of motion (ROM) and strength, complaint of pain, changes in sensation, balance and coordination status, and functional skill abilities. The goals of gait training may therefore be subdivided into the following major categories: general safety, decreased weight bearing, compensation for muscle weakness or loss of ROM, balance enhancement, and pain management (**Figure 4.1**). Once the goal of gait training is clearly understood, PTAs are able to take appropriate action in carrying out the plan of care. Clinical decisions are then based on an understanding of the patient's needs as well as his or her progress and performance.

◀ Attendance to the Rehabilitation Environment

A wide range of devices and equipment can be used to perform gait training. Plastic cones, rubber footprints, floor tape, as well as books and other general items may be used to fashion obstacle courses or guides for step-length or limb-shortening activities. Powdered chalk, black mats, stopwatches, and tape measures may be used to facilitate assessment of the objective parameters of gait. Assistive devices have varied features that allow for better patient customization (**Figure 4.2**). PTAs must know the benefits to using lofstrand versus axillary crutches or a standard walker versus a folding walker. A physical therapy clinic typically possesses a wide variety of gait aids. Often this equipment is neatly—or not so neatly—tucked away in closets and boxes.

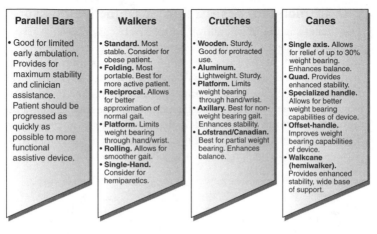

Parallel Bars	Walkers	Crutches	Canes
• Good for limited early ambulation. Provides for maximum stability and clinician assistance. Patient should be progressed as quickly as possible to more functional assistive device.	• **Standard.** Most stable. Consider for obese patient. • **Folding.** Most portable. Best for more active patient. • **Reciprocal.** Allows for better approximation of normal gait. • **Platform.** Limits weight bearing through hand/wrist. • **Rolling.** Allows for smoother gait. • **Single-Hand.** Consider for hemiparetics.	• **Wooden.** Sturdy. Good for protracted use. • **Aluminum.** Lightweight. Sturdy. • **Platform.** Limits weight bearing through hand/wrist. • **Axillary.** Best for non-weight bearing gait. Enhances stability. • **Lofstrand/Canadian.** Best for partial weight bearing. Enhances balance.	• **Single axis.** Allows for relief of up to 30% weight bearing. Enhances balance. • **Quad.** Provides enhanced stability. • **Specialized handle.** Allows for better weight bearing capabilities of device. • **Offset-handle.** Improves weight bearing capabilities of device. • **Walkcane (hemiwalker).** Provides enhanced stability, wide base of support.

Figure 4.2 Assistive Devices

PTAs must take special care to survey the available gait training equipment. By knowing what tools are available PTAs can better customize gait training to meet patients' needs.

◖ Understanding Patient/Family Needs

Clearly, an understanding of patient needs is crucial in gait training. For instance, a patient's pre-admission ambulation status will certainly affect clinical decision making. If a patient was a community ambulator without an assistive device prior to admission, the PTA may be more aggressive in progressing the patient to the least restrictive device. If the patient must climb several flights of stairs, the PTA may emphasize functional strengthening and ROM activities as part of the gait program. If a patient uses public transportation, high-stair climbing and endurance may be emphasized. PTAs must understand the gait needs of each patient. These needs may vary greatly from patient to patient. Rather than simply providing a cookie-cutter treatment progression, PTAs must strive to customize gait training to best meet each patient's needs.

◀ **Utilization and Assessment of Objective Measures**

The cyclical nature of gait allows for relatively easy objective assessment. Assessment of the objective measures of gait should serve as a basis for clinical decisions. Too often distance is used as the primary objective indicator, and goals are often written in terms of gait distance (e.g., "STG: Increase ambulation with walker to 60 feet"). However, more powerful and easily measured objective gait parameters exist. These measures include cadence, step length, and cycle time (**Figures 4.3** and **4.4**). Physical therapy clinicians should consider these parameters when making clinical decisions related to progression

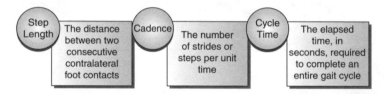

Figure 4.3 Easily Measured Objective Parameters of Gait

Step Length — The distance between two consecutive contralateral foot contacts

Cadence — The number of strides or steps per unit time

Cycle Time — The elapsed time, in seconds, required to complete an entire gait cycle

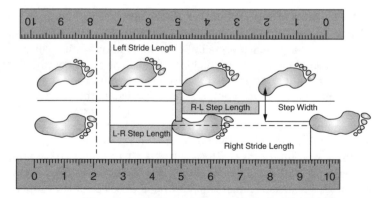

Left Stride Length
R-L Step Length
Step Width
L-R Step Length
Right Stride Length

Figure 4.4 Objective Spatial Parameters of Gait

and types of gait activities. For instance, normal gait is cyclical and relatively symmetrical. Asymmetry in right or left step times or step lengths is indicative of pathology (e.g., pain, ROM impairment, decreased muscle strength, etc.). Objective measurement of diminishing asymmetries, using simple tape measures and/or stopwatches, may influence clinical decisions. Such objective measurements may serve as the basis for progression and determining the effectiveness of the gait training (O'Sullivan & Schmitz, 2007).

While assessing patients' ambulation status, PTAs must assess and describe the assistance patients require. Too often, PTAs focus on the amount of assistance and not the reason that it is needed. A more complete description of the required level of assistance enhances clinical decision making. For example, it is not enough to say that a patient needs moderate assistance to ambulate with a walker. Why does the patient need moderate assistance? When does the patient need the assistance? Assistance may be required to move the walker forward, weight shift lower extremities, progress the weaker extremity, or to enhance balance. Answering these questions enhances clinical decision making.

When making a decision related to a patient's level of independence (e.g., contact guard, level of supervision, independence), PTAs need to ask themselves whether it is the patient who needs the assistance or if he or she feels the need to hold on to the patient. Novice PTAs, usually due to their own anxieties and inexperience, tend to not want to let go of their patients. They tend to overdocument that patients require contact guard. When making the clinical decision about levels of independence, PTAs must think about safety. Is the patient able to ambulate alone? In such instances it is helpful to ask, "If I left the room, would the patient be able to ambulate safely?"

◀ Progressive Ambulation Training with Assistive Devices

PTAs often have difficulty deciding when to progress a patient to the next least restrictive assistive device. This clinical decision is often based on several indicators, including the required level of assistance, functionality, gait distance, and efficiency. For instance, PTAs should

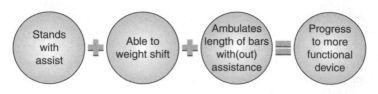

Figure 4.5 Factors Leading to Progressing Patient from Parallel Bars

strive to progress a patient from ambulation in parallel bars as quickly as possible. Though quite stable, the functionality of parallel bars is quite low. PTAs may ask a series of questions in deciding to progress the patient. Such questions may include: (1) Can the patient stand with assistance? (2) Is the patient able to weight shift? and (3) Can the patient ambulate the length of the bars (**Figure 4.5**)? Answering yes to these questions may lead PTAs to progress the patient to the next least restrictive device—a walker.

Effective progression requires continuous assessment. PTAs must constantly assess the effectiveness of the chosen assistive device. PTAs should seek answers to the following questions: Is the patient able to use the device correctly? Is the device giving the patient necessary support? Is the patient having the same ambulation problems as with the previous device or are there new problems? With practice, will the patient be able to ambulate independently with the device? The answers to these questions will help guide the decision making process (**Figures 4.6** and **4.7**).

◀ Possession of Sound Clinical Knowledge and Expertise

Gait is complex. Neuromuscular, musculoskeletal, and psychological factors affect gait. PTAs must understand how these factors influence clinical decision making. Rather than simply identifying phases of gait, PTAs must understand the goals of those phases and how, through muscle contraction, momentum, and joint mechanics, human locomotion is possible.

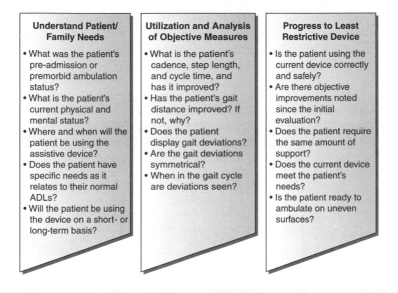

Understand Patient/Family Needs

- What was the patient's pre-admission or premorbid ambulation status?
- What is the patient's current physical and mental status?
- Where and when will the patient be using the assistive device?
- Does the patient have specific needs as it relates to their normal ADLs?
- Will the patient be using the device on a short- or long-term basis?

Utilization and Analysis of Objective Measures

- What is the patient's cadence, step length, and cycle time, and has it improved?
- Has the patient's gait distance improved? If not, why?
- Does the patient display gait deviations?
- Are the gait deviations symmetrical?
- When in the gait cycle are deviations seen?

Progress to Least Restrictive Device

- Is the patient using the current device correctly and safely?
- Are there objective improvements noted since the initial evaluation?
- Does the patient require the same amount of support?
- Does the current device meet the patient's needs?
- Is the patient ready to ambulate on uneven surfaces?

Figure 4.6 Clinical Decision-Making Factors in Gait Training

- Do activities address the patient's specific gait deviations?
- Have gait deviations improved? If not, why?
- Does the use of an assistive device alter the deviations?
- How is the patient's ambulation with respect to safety?
- Does the patient feel comfortable with the chosen assistive device?
- Has the patient made progress toward short- and long-term goals?

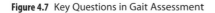

Figure 4.7 Key Questions in Gait Assessment

When pathology exists, PTAs must differentiate compensated and uncompensated deviations (**Figure 4.8**). For instance, if a patient displays hip hiking on the left side, the problem may derive from either the left or right side. The patient may be hiking the hip to compensate for a left foot drop or for a right hip abduction dysfunction. A better understanding as to what might be causing the deviation/compensation will affect clinical decision making (Skinner & Hurley, 2007). Whereas PTAs may not necessarily possess the full academic training to perform detailed gait analyses, they certainly should be able to recognize deviations from normal and consult a physical therapist.

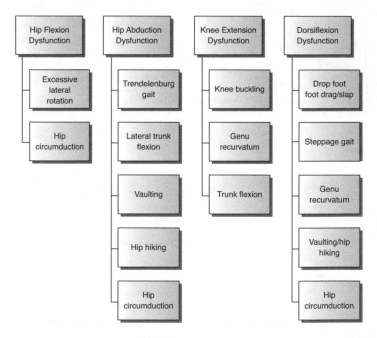

Figure 4.8 Common Gait Deviations and Compensations

◖ Limits on Clinical Decisions

Clear limits exist as to the types of clinical decisions PTAs may make with regard to gait training. Weight-bearing status is not open to interpretation. In cases where weight-bearing status is unclear, PTAs must consult a physical therapist for clarification. PTAs should not initiate orthotic use without first consulting a physical therapist. As with any case, major changes in a patient's ambulation status should be brought to the immediate attention of the supervising physical therapist for review and possible revision of the plan of care.

◖ References

O'Sullivan, S. B., & Schmitz, T. J. (2007). *Physical Rehabilitation* (5th ed.). Philadelphia, PA: F.A. Davis.

Skinner, S. B., & Hurley, C. (2007). *Pocket Notes for the Physical Therapist Assistant.* Sudbury, MA: Jones and Bartlett Publishers.

What Do YOU Think?

▶ **Scenario 1**

You are treating a 71-year-old patient who has just undergone a total knee arthroplasty (TKA) two days ago and is weight bearing as tolerated (WBAT) on his right lower extremity. The treatment plan includes therapeutic exercise, bed mobility, transfer, and progressive ambulation training. The therapist has started this patient ambulating with a standard walker.

   1. What gait pattern would be most appropriate for this patient and why?
   2. It is now four days later and the patient is ambulating independently with a standard walker over long distances. What assistive device can you try to progress this patient to? Justify your answer.

▶ **Scenario 2**

You are treating a 78-year-old patient who displays general deconditioning secondary to a prolonged hospitalization for multiple medical reasons. When you are ambulating this patient, you notice that the patient displays decreased heel strike bilaterally.

   1. What might be one possible cause of this decreased heel strike, and how might it be related to the patient's prolonged hospitalization?
   2. If the treatment plan for this patient included lower extremity exercises, what other type of exercise might this patient benefit from?

Level II Activity

▶ **Physical Therapy Evaluation**

Patient Name: _____

HPI: Pt. is a 75-year-old male s/p left THA last week secondary to OA. THA surgery was done by an anterior approach. Pt. is WBAT on the left LE. Pt. was admitted to this inpatient rehab. center on post-op day 5. Pt. is being seen for PT.

PMH: HTN, OA throughout, right TKA

MEDS: Cardizem, Percocet

SH: Pt. lives alone in an apartment with 12 steps to enter. Stairs have a railing on the right side. Prior to admission, pt. was independent in ADLs and amb. with a straight cane.

Mental Status: Pt. is alert and oriented × 3. Pt. is able to follow commands without difficulty.

ROM: Bilateral UE and LE are WFL throughout except right knee flex/ext 0-100 degrees and left hip flex. 0–70 degrees, abd. 0–15 degrees. IR/ER and hip ext not assessed due to pt.'s pain.

Muscle Strength: Bilateral UE and LE are G throughout except left hip not fully assessed secondary to pain.

Sensation: Pt.'s sensation to light touch is intact throughout.

Pain: Pt. complains of mild joint stiffness throughout. Pt. complains of pain in the left hip with movement, 6/10 on the pain scale.

Muscle Tone: Pt. displays no abnormal muscle tone.

Balance: Sitting balance—normal. Standing—pt. is able to stand with CG.

Functional Status: Pt. is able to roll to the left with min. assist. Pt. transfers supine ←→ sit with mod. assist, sit ←→ stand with mod. assist. Pt. amb. with left LE WBAT with walker for 10 feet with mod. assist. Pt. is very hesitant to WB on left LE.

Problems: Pain, decreased active movement, decreased strength, decreased balance, dependency in functional skills.

Short-Term Goals: Pt.'s left hip ROM will increase 10 degrees. Pt. will transfer supine ←→ sit with CG and sit ←→ stand with min. assist. Pt. will amb. with the appropriate assistive device 100 feet with min. assist for balance and weight shifting. Pt. will be independent in TH precautions.

Long-Term Goals: Pt. will be independent in transfers. Pt. will ambulate with an appropriate assist device with supervision on level surfaces and on stairs.

Assessment: Pt. is motivated and very cooperative. Pt. appears to be a good rehab. candidate.

Plan: Daily PT for therapeutic exercise, bed mobility, transfers, and ambulation training.

Precautions: THA precautions

Activity: Mr. Brown was evaluated last week and has been treated by a physical therapist since the evaluation. The patient is now ambulating with a walker for 100 feet with supervision with left LE WBAT and will be discharged in two days. Today the PT has asked you to treat this patient. After the treatment is completed, write a progress note and answer the following questions.

1. What assistive device did you use with this patient today and why?
2. What type of gait pattern did you instruct this patient to use and why?
3. What treatment did you do with this patient today to prepare him for discharge?

Clinical Decision Making in Administering Thermal Modalities

If a modality is used to manage pain, then pain assessments should be performed immediately following its administration. If used to reduce spasms, then post-treatment palpation, active ROM, or other assessments should be performed. Effectiveness helps drive clinical decisions. To ensure effective implementation of the plan of care, PTAs must always strive to utilize all objective assessments. Assessment of a modality's effectiveness should always be a routine aspect of physical therapy intervention.

Thermal agents are probably the most often used modalities in physical therapy. They play a major adjunctive role in the overall plan of care. Given the ubiquity and seemingly casual use of these modalities, PTAs may mistakenly apply them with less critical thought. PTAs must guard against simply slapping on a hot pack or haphazardly applying ultrasound. They must make critical and well thought out clinical decisions related to selection, placement, and application of these important modalities.

◀ Goals of Treatment

When administering a thermal modality, PTAs must clearly understand the reasons for its use. Understanding the intended goals for the use of the modality significantly influences clinical decisions related to how and when the modality is applied. For instance, say that a PTA is assigned a patient with a diagnosis of right shoulder adhesive capsulitis. The plan of care includes (1) hot packs, (2) ultrasound, (3) cryotherapy, (4) PROM activities, and (5) AROM activities. Generally,

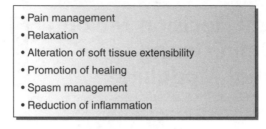

- Pain management
- Relaxation
- Alteration of soft tissue extensibility
- Promotion of healing
- Spasm management
- Reduction of inflammation

Figure 5.1 Common Goals of Thermotherapy

the goals of thermal modalities include pain management, relaxation, alteration of soft tissue extensibility, promotion of healing, spasm management, and reduction of inflammation (**Figure 5.1**). These are all potential goals in the management of adhesive capsulitis. If the primary goal for the use of heat is to manage pain, PTAs must make critical decisions related to pre- and post-intervention assessment and modality placement. If the primary goal is to increase tissue extensibility, the PTA must make the clinical decision to administer stretching and ROM activities at the appropriate time in order to maximize the effects of tissue heating.

As with all interventions, when considering the use of thermal modalities PTAs must take special care to recognize the prescribed goals. Sometimes these goals may not be specifically tied to the prescribed modality. Ideally, the initial evaluation may state "moist heat for pain management"; however, sometimes the prescribed modalities and selected intervention goals are documented in separate lists. PTAs may then need to rely upon their knowledge of the physiological effects of thermal modalities in order to match the appropriate modality with the intended goal. The more complex the case, the more prescriptive and exact the plan of care and goals are likely to be. In these cases, PTAs may more easily implement the plan of care as written. However, in less complex cases PTs may assume that PTAs have the appropriate clinical and academic training to make the appropriate clinical decisions and render effective physical therapy care. Whether involved in managing simple or complex cases,

PTAs must be very aware of therapeutic goals and from that awareness make effective clinical decisions.

◀ Attendance to the Rehabilitation Environment

Several common therapeutic thermal modalities are available (**Figure 5.2**). Most often, PTAs are not required to make clinical decisions related to the selection of a particular modality. Physical therapists specify which thermal modalities are to be administered. As it relates to clinical decision making in administering thermal modalities, attendance to the rehabilitation environment is more so associated with PTAs' abilities to discern use patterns, equipment availability, and alternatives.

Given their ease of use, ability to heat tissue, and relatively low costs, hot packs are likely the most often used—perhaps overused—thermal modality. In very busy clinics, hot packs are removed from the heating unit, cooled during patient use, and placed back into the heating unit at continuous and regular intervals. Typically, once cooled a hot pack requires at least 20 minutes of submersion in the heating unit to reach therapeutic temperatures (Behrens & Michlovitz, 2006, p. 42).

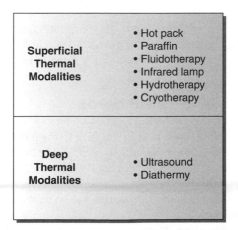

Superficial Thermal Modalities	• Hot pack • Paraffin • Fluidotherapy • Infrared lamp • Hydrotherapy • Cryotherapy
Deep Thermal Modalities	• Ultrasound • Diathermy

Figure 5.2 Common Thermal Modalities

During peak usage times, hot packs may be repeatedly removed and used before reaching therapeutic temperatures.

If PTAs are aware of such usage patterns, they may make various clinical decisions to attempt to maximize effectiveness. The ideal decision is to suggest to the supervising physical therapist the purchasing of additional hot packs and heating units. To better enhance heat transfer, PTAs may also decide to cautiously reduce the layers of toweling between the hot pack and the patient's skin. Such clinical decisions are made based upon the recognition of potential inadequacies in the rehabilitation environment and the understanding that for a hot pack to be therapeutic sufficient heat energy must be transferred. An insufficient transfer of heat energy certainly hampers goal attainment.

PTAs may make clinical decisions related to how a particular thermal modality is applied. For instance, given the severity of inflammation, PTAs make a clinical decision to use a cold pack versus an ice pack. The ice pack most likely results in a more significant and rapid transfer of heat, which is more desirable in managing severe or acute inflammation (Michlovitz & Nolan, 2005). When inflammation around a joint is particularly acute, PTAs may make the clinical decision to seek approval for use of a device that combines compression and cryotherapy. In both of these instances, the goal of the cryotherapy is to manage inflammation. However, by attending to the rehabilitation environment—recognizing the available clinical means to accomplish goals—PTAs may be able to better tailor interventions to patients' immediate clinical condition.

◀ Understanding Patient Needs

When administering thermal modalities, understanding patient needs is primarily associated with being sensitive to the patient's safety and comfort. These needs are related to patient perception/sensation, the presence of contraindications, and the recognition of treatment precautions (**Figure 5.3**). For instance, when treating severe inflammation PTAs may make the clinical decision to use an ice pack rather than a gel-based cold pack. However, if the patient is unable to tolerate the relative increased intensity of the ice pack a decision to use the cold pack may be made.

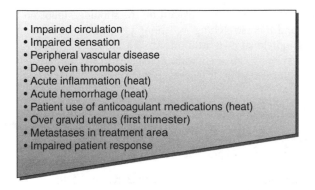

- Impaired circulation
- Impaired sensation
- Peripheral vascular disease
- Deep vein thrombosis
- Acute inflammation (heat)
- Acute hemorrhage (heat)
- Patient use of anticoagulant medications (heat)
- Over gravid uterus (first trimester)
- Metastases in treatment area
- Impaired patient response

Figure 5.3 General Contraindications and Precautions for Thermal Modalities

Respiratory problems or obesity may prevent a patient with low back pain from comfortably assuming the prone position. The prone position is ideal when applying a hot pack to the low back. In the presence of obesity, respiratory, or other position limiting factors, PTAs may make the clinical decision to suggest an alternative means of delivering moist heat. For instance PTAs may suggest the use of an infrared lamp and moist toweling to deliver heat energy. The use of infrared may negate the need to assume the prone position. With infrared, heat might be able to be administered in a side lying or even a modified sitting position more safely than with a hot pack. Making decisions that reflect understanding of patients' immediate clinical needs helps insure effective and safe delivery of thermal modalities (Prentice, 2005).

◀ Utilization and Assessment of Objective Measures

PTAs must be able to assess the effectiveness of the various thermal modalities. As previously stated, thermal therapy has several goals (Figure 5.1). Sometimes thermal modalities are seemingly applied simply as routine prerequisites for later interventions—without appropriate care or forethought. Unfortunately, these modalities are sometimes used more as convenient time-management tools. Oftentimes effectiveness is assumed—a hot pack is placed on the shoulder, followed by ultra-sound, and then stretching—without a real effort to assess effectiveness of individual goal attainment. If a modality is used to manage pain, then pain assessments should be performed immediately following its administration. If used to reduce spasms, then post-treatment palpation, active ROM, or other assessments should be performed. Effectiveness helps drive clinical decisions. To ensure effective implementation of the plan of care, PTAs must always strive to utilize all objective assessments. Assessment of a modality's effectiveness should always be a routine aspect of physical therapy intervention.

◀ Possession of Sound Clinical Knowledge and Expertise

When making clinical decisions about administering thermal modalities, PTAs must rely on sound clinical knowledge and expertise. First and foremost, PTAs must possess the appropriate knowledge and expertise to make sound clinical decisions related to patient safety. They must be vigilant in detecting contraindications and precautions. For instance, an episodic acute joint inflammation precludes the use of heat. Sound clinical knowledge and expertise demand careful pre and post inspection of the treatment area. Such inspections lead to clinical decisions related to potential changes in how or if modalities are applied.

As previously stated, in certain clinical situations heating with an infrared lamp may be substituted for hot packs. However, PTAs must know that the depth of penetration from the infrared lamp is much less than with a hot pack and that additional safety precautions must be considered (**Figure 5.4**). Before suggesting this substitution, PTAs must decide whether the trade-off in depth of penetration will still facilitate goal attainment.

Similarly, when a patient presents with signs of overdosage of ultrasound, PTAs correctly make the clinical decision to lower the dosage. However, PTAs should understand that in order to achieve the desired level of heating, decreased intensity must be accompanied by increased treatment time. If treatment dosage is decreased by a third, treatment time should be increased by at least the same proportion.

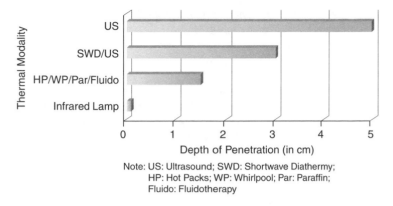

Note: US: Ultrasound; SWD: Shortwave Diathermy;
HP: Hot Packs; WP: Whirlpool; Par: Paraffin;
Fluido: Fluidotherapy

Figure 5.4 Depth of Penetration for Common Thermal Modalities

This clinical decision is made based on a thorough understanding of the administration of therapeutic ultrasound. Ultrasound may be prescribed for the management of a supraspinatus tendon tear. The dosage and treatment time is determined by PTs based on the size of the treatment area and other factors. Physical therapists must have confidence in PTAs' sound knowledge of anatomy. Ultrasound to the supraspinatus tendon does not mean that ultrasound is applied to the shoulder region. To be effective, the sonic waves must be directed at the target tissue. This understanding helps to drive clinical decisions related to patient positioning and delivery techniques.

When administering heat, PTAs must make sound time-management and patient-positioning decisions. Heat decreases viscosity and increases extensibility of connective tissue. These physiological effects greatly contribute to increases in range of motion with heat application. However, PTAs must be mindful that heated connective tissue is most extensible while being vigorously heated and that it cools relatively quickly following heating. When using heat to increase range of motion, PTAs should make the decision to position the joint so that target structures are on slight stretch. Further, PTAs must be prepared to perform stretching and other ROM activities immediately following the heat treatment. These considerations may not be explicitly detailed in the formal plan of care. Physical therapists may assume that by virtue of their training PTAs possess the appropriate knowledge and expertise to make appropriate clinical decisions to increase the probability of goal achievement.

◀ Limits on Clinical Decisions

As it relates to some thermal modalities, physical therapists' plans of care tend to be quite prescriptive. For example, dosage, frequency, and duration in administering ultrasound are clearly prescribed. Generally, PTAs may not decide to change these parameters without physical therapist consent.

◀ References

Behrens, B. J., & Michlovitz, S. L. (2006). *Physical Agents: Theory and Practice* (2nd ed.). Philadelphia, PA: F.A. Davis.

Michlovitz, S. L., & Nolan, T. P. (2005). *Modalities for Therapeutic Intervention.* Philadelphia, PA: F.A. Davis.

Prentice, W. E. (2005). *Therapeutic Modalities in Rehabilitation* (3rd ed.). New York: McGraw-Hill.

What Do YOU Think?

▶ **Scenario 1 (Level I)**

You are treating a patient who is suffering from low back pain. As part of the treatment you give this patient a hot pack.

1. After 5 minutes, the patient complains that the hot pack is getting too hot. What do you do? What might be the cause of the patient's discomfort?
2. Following treatment, the patient presents with physical signs of overheating. Describe those signs. What clinical decisions would you make as a result of your observations?

▶ **Scenario 2 (Level II)**

You are treating a patient who is suffering from bicipital tendonitis. As part of the treatment, you give this patient ultrasound to her shoulder.

1. The patient asks you why she cannot feel anything during the ultrasound. What do you say?
2. You are treating another patient with the same diagnosis. Only this patient complains of heat when receiving ultrasound. Why might this be happening?

Level I Activity

▶ **Physical Therapy Evaluation**

Patient Name: _____

Diagnosis: Adhesive capsulitis left shoulder

History: Patient is a 53-year-old male who presents with a chief complaint of left shoulder pain and stiffness. The patient states that he has had increased symptoms in the last two weeks following raking leaves outside. He began having intermittent pain two years ago following continuous overhead activities. Patient states that the pain is "not bad" now, but he notes that it has begun to worsen. He describes the pain as a "tightness with activities" with occasional morning "numbness" of the left arm. Pain is 5/10 in the left shoulder with overhead activities.

Objective Findings: Inspection reveals no major asymmetries. Palpation is negative for pain or abnormality. Range of motion at the left shoulder reveals 0–120 degrees of abduction, 0–140 degrees of flexion, 0–20 degrees of external rotation, and normal internal rotation. Patient has pain at the end ranges of all movements. End feel for all movements is capsular. Strength of the left shoulder is generally graded as 3/5 and 5/5 on the right.

Resisted movements do not reproduce pain. Cervical nerve root strength tests are negative for weakness. Cervical range of motion is within normal limits. Deep tendon reflexes are present and equal bilaterally.

Assessment: Patient presents with signs and symptoms consistent with an adhesive capsulitis, as evidenced by a capsular pattern of tightness at the left shoulder. Some weakness of the left shoulder muscles is also noted. The patient would benefit from physical therapy for restoration of normal shoulder range of motion and strengthening activities.

Goals: STG: ROM of the left shoulder will increase 10 degrees in order to perform overhead activities. Pt.'s pain will decrease to 3–4/10 on pain scale in order to perform more functional skills.

LTG: Left shoulder ROM will be WNL. Pt.'s strength of left shoulder will be 4+/5 and patient will be independent in UE functional activities.

Plan: Physical therapy two times weekly for four weeks for thermal modalities, passive stretching, electrical stimulation, home exercise program.

Instructions: The physical therapist completed the above evaluation yesterday and has asked you to treat this patient today. After completing the treatment answer the following questions.
1. What thermal activities would be most appropriate for this patient and why?
2. Where within the treatment would you place these modalities and why?

Level II Activity

▶ **Physical Therapy Evaluation**
Patient Name: _____

Diagnosis: Cervical pain secondary to motor vehicle accident

HPI: The patient is a 43-year-old female who was involved in a motor vehicle accident one month ago. The patient states that one week after the accident she was unable to move the left shoulder and that she had neck, chest, and back pain. X-rays at the hospital were negative for fractures/dislocations. The patient is currently complaining of neck pain, 7/10 on pain scale with movement, especially rotation.

Objective Findings: Inspection of the cervical region reveals a slightly reduced cervical lordosis. Bilateral medial winging of scapulae is noted. No gross asymmetries noted. Palpation is negative. Moderate to severe limitation in cervical rotation noted. The patient is unable to look over either shoulder. Side flexion and cervical flexion presents with moderate limitations. Pain is noted at the end ranges of all cervical movements. Passive cervical movements present with the same limitations as active movements. Cervical nerve root strength tests are negative for weakness. Deep tendon reflexes are equal and present bilaterally. Sensation to pin prick and light touch is intact.

Assessment: Patient presents with significantly decreased cervical range of motion. Cervical range of motion is limited passively as well as actively. This may suggest significant soft tissue shortening. There does not appear to be any significant neurological deficits. The patient may benefit from physical therapy to restore cervical range of motion, restore anatomical alignment, and decrease cervical pain.

Goals: STG: Increase cervical rotation, pt. will be able to look over either shoulder. Pt. will be able to perform side flexion and cervical flexion without pain.

LTG: Pt.'s cervical ROM will be WNL.

Plan: Physical therapy twice weekly for six weeks for hot pack, ultrasound, electric stimulation, ROM activities, and home exercise program.

Instructions: The physical therapist completed this evaluation yesterday and has asked you to treat this patient today. Based on this evaluation, answer the following questions.

1. What would be the treatment rationale for giving this patient ultrasound?
2. How might these modalities be strategically placed to best benefit this patient?
3. How could have the PT evaluation have better assisted you in gauging progress?

Clinical Decision Making in Administering Electrical Stimulation

Although some evidence suggests that acute and musculoskeletal problems respond better to gate control strategies and that chronic sharp pain responds more to central biasing strategies, if not specified by the PT, the results should guide the application of the theories. For example, if a patient is not responding to electrical stimulation, as evidenced by a lack demonstrable pain relief as indicated on a visual analog scale), the PTA may decide to change the parameters of the electrical stimulation consistent with an alternate theory.

The use of electrical stimulation in physical therapy provides many physiological benefits, and a variety of clinical decisions can enhance its effectiveness. PTAs must be aware of the various electrical stimulation parameters, including goals, waveform, electrode placement, frequency, and others. Clearly, electrical stimulation is much more than simply slapping on a couple of electrodes and turning up the juice. Great care must be taken to ensure that the appropriate parameters are matched to patients' conditions, responses, and therapeutic goals.

This chapter discusses and presents various factors that influence clinical decision making in electrical stimulation. Note, however, that it is beyond the scope of this text to provide detailed didactic information related to electrical stimulation. This type of information can be found in several other published texts. Instead, this chapter will focus on the general processes required to make sound clinical decisions.

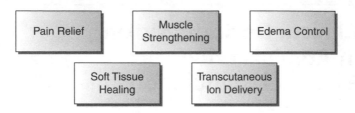

Figure 6.1 Major Therapeutic Goals for the Use of Electrical Stimulation

◀ Goals of Electrical Stimulation

It is crucial that PTAs know why electrical stimulation has been included in a plan of care. The initial evaluation should clearly delineate the goals of electrical stimulation. Goals of electrical stimulation will surely influence all subsequent clinical decisions. Electrical stimulation goals can easily be subdivided into the following major categories: pain relief, muscle strengthening/reeducation, edema control, facilitation of soft tissue healing, and transcutaneous delivery of therapeutic ions (**Figure 6.1**). These goals dictate the type of electrical stimulation administered.

◀ Attendance to the Rehabilitation Environment

Although the same electrical stimulator may be used to treat a variety of conditions, the parameters for pain relief differ greatly from the parameters for edema control or muscle strengthening/reeducation.

Conversely, some electrical stimulators can only be used to achieve a single therapeutic goal (e.g., a TENS unit for pain relief). It is important that PTAs carefully survey the electrical stimulation equipment at their disposal. For instance, they must know which machines are high voltage or low voltage, which machines allow for pulse duration (width) alteration, or which ones allow for variable ramp/surge settings. Rather than selecting equipment based on availability, clinician comfort level, or some other personal preference, PTAs should always choose the equipment that best matches the therapeutic goals.

◀ Understanding Patient/Family Needs

It is also important to understand patient needs when administering electrical stimulation. For example, a relatively active patient with mild-to-moderate low back pain may benefit from immediate use of TENS (transcutaneous electrical nerve stimulation) for pain relief. A TENS effect may be administered via an ambulatory TENS unit or a table model electrical stimulator. When using a TENS unit, part of the treatment session may be more active. The patient may perform work activities and activities of daily living while receiving the TENS. Early use of TENS will allow for an effective evaluation of its efficacy. In contrast, a more sedentary patient with moderate-to-severe low back pain may benefit from a combination of moist heat and electrical stimulation in the prone position. If treating an injured athlete for muscle strengthening, a home stimulator may be appropriate. An athlete may have a need to regain strength at a faster pace than a nonathlete. Clearly, these scenarios require PTAs to understand the needs and goals of the patient. The electrotherapy must be tailored to the patient's needs.

◀ Utilization and Assessment of Objective Measures

When making clinical decisions related to administering electrical stimulation, PTAs must rely on the use and assessment of objective measures. When managing pain, PTAs must make judicious use of visual analog scales and pain questionnaires. Manual muscle testing, dynametrics, and functional tests can be used to monitor strength gains. Circumferential and volumetric measurements can be used for effective monitoring of changes in edema. Portable digitizers, digital cameras, and flexible rulers can be used to monitor size changes in open wounds. The data collected using these and other objective tools provide the necessary cues for the required gross or subtle changes in electrical stimulation parameters.

◀ Possession of Sound Clinical Knowledge and Expertise

PTAs' clinical knowledge and expertise is crucial to the effective administration of electrotherapy. Electrical stimulation alters cellular physiology. PTAs must understand the underlying physiology and the therapeutic benefits. They must be able to relate the various stimulation parameters to the physiological results and manipulate them accordingly. The following paragraphs will examine the type of clinical knowledge required in order to administer sound electrotherapy.

◖ Electrical Stimulation for Pain Management

The main theories that support the use of electrical stimulation in pain management are the gate control theory, the central biasing theory, and the endogenous opiate theory. **Figure 6.2** briefly describes these theories and the electrical stimulation parameters associated with each (Prentice, 2005). Although some evidence suggests that acute and musculoskeletal problems respond better to gate control

Gate Control Theory	Central Biasing Theory	Endogenous Opiate Theory
Sensory stimulation of sensory alpha beta fibers block the gate of pain in the substantia gelatinosa of the dorsal horn of the spinal cord. Requires pulse width of 75–150 microseconds and a frequency of 80–125 pps.	Intense short-term stimulation of small C fibers at trigger or acupuncture points lead to the firing of descending central fibers that close the gate for pain in the substantia gelatinosa region of the spinal cord. Requires a pulse width of about 10 milliseconds, a frequency of 80 pps, and an on-time of 30 seconds to 1 minute.	Intense sensory stimulation of sensory nerves may stimulate the release of endogenous opiates from the central nervous system with resulting circulation in the cerebral spinal fluid. Electrical stimulation is applied with a point stimulator and large dispersive pad near the site of pain or at trigger or acupuncture points. Intensity should be high, pulse duration between 200 microseconds to 10 milliseconds, and a frequency of 1–5 pps. An on-time of 30–45 seconds is best.

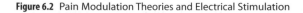

Figure 6.2 Pain Modulation Theories and Electrical Stimulation

strategies and that chronic sharp pain responds more to central biasing strategies, if not specified by the PT, the results should guide the application of the theories. For example, if a patient is not responding to electrical stimulation, as evidenced by a lack of demonstrable pain relief as indicated on a visual analog scale), the PTA may decide to change the parameters of the electrical stimulation consistent with an alternate theory.

When applying the gate control theory, PTAs may vary electrode placement. Effectiveness of pain relief may be enhanced by simply altering electrode placement. PTAs should not haphazardly place electrodes. Placement should be based on clinical and academic knowledge and carefully documented. When desired results are not achieved, PTAs may change the electrode placement. **Figure 6.3** describes some electrode placement options. PTAs must remember that therapeutic benefits of electrical stimulation for pain relief may be evidenced as soon as the initial intervention. By carefully monitoring patient response, PTAs may make sound clinical decisions to achieve therapeutic goals.

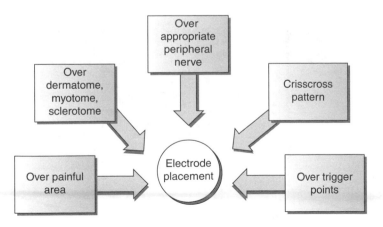

Figure 6.3 Popular Electrode Placement Options for Pain Management

◖ Electrical Stimulation to Facilitate Muscle Contraction

Whether using electrical stimulation to facilitate muscle pumping to manage edema or for muscle strengthening/reeducation, PTAs can make several clinical decisions to enhance its effectiveness. Primary concerns when administering this type of intervention are quality of muscle contraction and patient comfort. PTAs often make clinical decisions concerning ramp time, pulse duration, and frequency. These electrical stimulation parameters significantly influence effectiveness. Further, PTAs may also have the opportunity to determine whether a bipolar or monopolar technique is preferable. Once again, it should be stated that these parameters (**Figure 6.4**) may indeed be specified by the physical therapist. Absent specification by the physical therapist, PTAs must possess the basic clinical skills necessary to effectively manage these parameters in reaction to patient response. For example, therapeutic muscle contraction requires a certain stimulus intensity. However, when the PTA achieves this intensity the patient may

Ramp/Surge	Pulse Width	Frequency	Bipolar vs. Monopolar
Ramp controls the rate of rise of the electrical stimulus. A slower ramp time may more closely mimic recruitment patterns and may enhance comfort.	Pulse width refers to the duration of the stimulus. Many low-volt stimulators allow for adjustment of pulse width. Longer pulse widths may enhance contraction without increasing intensity, thereby enhancing comfort.	Frequency refers to the number of electrical impulses generated per second. A smooth tetanic contraction is required for muscle strengthening. A series of stronger twitch-type contractions are appropriate for edema management. The lowest possible frequency to achieve desired results should be used.	A bipolar technique uses same-sized active and dispersive pads. It is primarily used for the stimulation of large muscle groups. A monopolar technique uses a small active electrode or probe and a distal large dispersive pad. It is used to stimulate smaller individual muscles.

Figure 6.4 Electrical Stimulation Parameters Critical to Facilitation of Muscle Contraction

complain of discomfort. If the PTA only decreases the intensity, the discomfort may lessen, but the desired contraction is lost. Instead, the PTA should decrease the intensity slightly and increase the pulse duration. This may preserve the contractile response and lessen the discomfort (Skinner & Hurley, 2007). Other parameters, such as duty cycle (on/off times) and electrode placement also require sound clinical decisions. For instance, PTAs must remember that due to repeated stimulation of the same motor units, electrically stimulated muscle tends to fatigue more quickly than normally contracting muscle. Alteration of duty cycle by increasing the time between contractions may help prevent excessive fatigue (Behrens & Michlovitz, 2006).

◀ Limits on Clinical Decisions

Just because PTAs may make a wide variety of clinical decisions related to the administration of electrical stimulation does not mean that they must. Indeed, PTAs must follow the parameters and techniques as specifically detailed by the physical therapist. If such specification is missing, PTAs must obtain the appropriate information prior to administering treatment—indeed, a prudent clinical decision. For example, when administering iontophoresis PTAs can manipulate intensity to enhance patient comfort (with appropriate adjustment of treatment time). However, the physical therapist's specification of ionic agent, polarity, and dosage must be followed without variation. Similarly, if the plan of care calls for low-voltage direct current to stimulate denervated muscle, PTAs may not substitute high-voltage or AC stimulation—even if they do enhance patient comfort.

PTAs' clinical decisions must always be made in the best interest of the patient. Any time the PTA is uncomfortable making a clinical decision, the PTA must seek guidance from a physical therapist.

◀ References

Behrens, B. J., & Michlovitz, S. L. (2006). *Physical Agents: Theory and Practice* (2nd ed.). Philadelphia, PA: F.A. Davis.

Prentice, W. E. (2005). *Therapeutic Modalities in Rehabilitation* (3rd ed.). New York: McGraw-Hill.

Skinner, S. B., & Hurley, C. (2007). *Pocket Notes for the Physical Therapist Assistant.* Sudbury, MA: Jones and Bartlett Publishers.

What Do YOU Think?

▶ **Scenario 1 (Level I)**

You are treating a patient with a diagnosis of bulging lumbar disc resulting in pain with flexion activities. The treatment plan calls for thermal modalities, electrical stimulation, passive lumbar extension exercises, and good body mechanic education. Your patient enters therapy today and says his pain is 6/10 on a pain scale. During the patient's treatment today, when would you give this patient electric stimulation?

▶ **Scenario 2 (Level II)**

You are treating a patient with a quadriceps tendon rupture. The treatment plan calls for electrical stimulation for muscle reeducation. What type of electrical stimulation would you use and how might you combine the stimulation with exercise?

Level I Activity

▶ **Physical Therapy Evaluation**

Patient Name: _____

History: Patient is a 32-year-old male with a diagnosis of acute low back pain secondary to a lifting injury two weeks ago.

PMH: Inguinal hernia repair six years ago.

SH: Pt. works as a driver/deliverer for a trucking company. Lives with wife and two small children.

Mental Status: Pt. is A&O × 3.

ROM: Lumbar ROM is moderately limited in all directions due to pain.

Strength: Good strength right UE and LE

Functional: Pt. has difficulty moving from sit to stand and bed mobility due to complaint of sharp pain with these activities. Pt. complains of constant low back ache that limits all activities. Pt. is unable to perform full work responsibilities due to pain at the left lower lumbar region.

Problems: (1) Loss of lumbar ROM, (2) low back pain, and (3) decreased work/ADL capabilities.

Goals: STG: Improve lumbar ROM, decrease low back pain, improve ADL.

LTG: Restore to normal pain-free function.

Treatment Plan: Conventional TENS, moist heat, lumbar ROM activities, postural retraining, body mechanic training

Activity: On his initial treatment session, the PTA sets the patient up with TENS as prescribed. During the treatment the patient states there is no change in his pain.

1. What are the likely TENS parameters selected by the PTA?
2. What actions might the PTA take to address the patient's report of no change in his pain?

Level II Activity

▶ **Physical Therapy Evaluation**
Patient Name: _____

History: Patient is a 20-year-old collegiate soccer player s/p left mid-tibia multiple stress fractures. Patient has been ambulating partial weight bearing with an ischial weight-bearing orthosis and axillary crutches for 10 weeks. Patient is now ambulating with a standard cane without orthosis. Patient states the cane is now being used for safety.

PMH: Right grade I knee MCL sprain two years ago.

SH: Lives at home with parents. Pt. commutes to college.

Mental Status: Pt. is A&O × 3.

ROM: ROM at all UE and LE joints is WNL.

Strength: Left quadriceps and hamstring strength is F+. Adductor strength is F+ and abductor strength is G.

Functional: Pt. ambulates independently with straight cane. Decreased step length on right is noted. Patient complains of left LE fatigue and knee buckling after walking moderate distances. Pt. is independent in all transfers and ADLs.

Problems: (1) Decreased left quad/ham and adductor strength, (2) left LE muscular fatigue, (3) ambulation with cane.

Goals: STG: Increase left LE muscle strength by half a grade; improve endurance. LTG: Improve left LE muscle strength to N throughout; improve endurance to athletic grade; return to athletic activity.

Treatment Plan: Electrical stimulation for muscle strengthening, progressive resistive exercises, endurance-training activities.

Activity: On his initial treatment session, the PTA sets the patient up with quadriceps-strengthening exercises with simultaneous electrical stimulation.

1. Was a bipolar or monopolar technique likely used? Describe the selected technique.
2. If the patient complained of excessive fatigue during simultaneous electrical stimulation and exercise, what clinical decision might the PTA make to address the issue?

Level II Activity

▶ **Physical Therapy Evaluation**
Patient Name: _____

HPI: Patient is a 42-year-old obese female who presents with severe edema of left leg secondary to chronic venous insufficiency.

PMH: Patient presents with HTN and hyperglycemia.

SH: Lives with husband and teenage daughter in two-story private home. She works as an administrative assistant. Currently she is not working and is receiving short-term disability benefits.

Mental Status: Pt. is A&O × 3.

ROM: Left ankle dorsiflexion ROM is 0–8 degrees, plantar flexion is 0–20 degrees. Edema appears to be the limiting ROM factor. Knee ROM is WFL and hip ROM is WNL.

Strength: Dorsiflexor strength is F and plantar flexor strength is F+.

Functional: Pt. ambulates short distances with a straight cane. She has difficulty negotiating stairs. She complains of fatigue and leg pain with activity.

Problems: (1) Left leg edema (2) Decreased ROM at left knee and ankle (3) Decreased strength left plantar/dorsiflexors

Goals: STG: Reduce edema by 3 cm; improve strength by one half grade; improve ROM by 6 degrees.

LTG: Control/maintain edema within 10% of uninvolved extremity; improve/maintain dorsi/plantar/flexor strength to G/N; improve endurance and ADL.

Treatment Plan: Electrical stimulation for edema control, intermittent compression therapy, progressive resistive exercises, ROM activities, endurance-training activities.

Activity: On the initial treatment session the PTA administers electrical stimulation with elevation in an attempt to decrease the edema.
1. What would be the best way to monitor the edema and assess the efficacy of the treatment?
2. Which muscles were likely targeted during the electrical stimulation?
3. Would a monopolar or bipolar technique be used?
4. What would be a likely pulse frequency?

Clinical Decision Making in Managing Neurological (CNS) Conditions

PTAs must be ever ready to receive, process, and incorporate new knowledge into their clinical arsenal. When confronted with less familiar clinical scenarios, reviewing and refreshing of concepts and facts should be the order of the day. PTAs must embrace the notion that there is always more to learn and always a means to enhance treatment efficacy, thus maintaining an inquisitive clinical demeanor.

Sequelae is a medical term used to describe the secondary after-effects of disease. Neurological conditions are often characterized by significant multiple sequelae. These sequelae influence rehabilitation and clinical decision making (**Figure 7.1**). When carrying out treatment plans and making clinical decisions, PTAs must identify, sort, and prioritize these sequelae. Effective PTAs do not simply perform a set of PT prescribed interventions. Instead, they fashion those prescribed interventions into a coherent and logical treatment sequence that best meet the rehabilitation goals. This requires PTAs to make clinical decisions based on a clear understanding of the condition and the various factors that influence rehabilitation.

◀ Goals of Treatment

As a result of multiple sequelae, the management of neurological conditions often includes the setting of several treatment goals. For instance, an initial evaluation for a patient with CVA, multiple sclerosis (MS), or traumatic brain injury (TBI) may include goals that address ambulation,

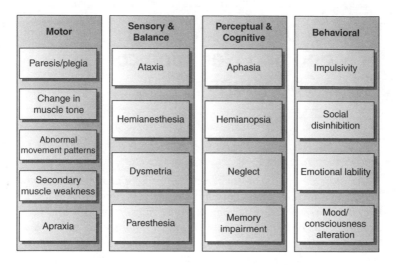

Figure 7.1 Common Sequelae Associated with Neurological Disorders

transfers, muscle tone, activities of daily living, general movement patterns, and perceptual compensations. These goals are often presented in a list; each standing distinctly alone. Whereas this listing is crucial for literary clarity and for third-party payment consideration, PTAs must be able to clearly discern how the goals interact with one another. Can ambulation training effectively proceed if muscle tone is not addressed? Can a patient progress to supervised transfers if interventions to address unilateral neglect are not initiated? Can activities of daily living improve if volitional movement is too heavily influenced by mass patterns? Indeed, treatment goals never stand alone. They must be seen in the context of the entire clinical picture. The most effective PTAs prioritize treatment goals in recognition of the sequelae's cascading affects (**Figure 7.2**). Once understood and appropriately prioritized, the goals will help guide clinical decisions. Such decisions include selection of specific interventions, the sequence of interventions, and a determination of self-management strategies.

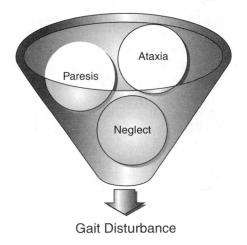

Gait Disturbance

Figure 7.2 Cascading Effect of Common Sequelae

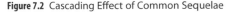

◀ Attendance to the Rehabilitation Environment

When managing neurological disorders, PTAs are often limited only by their imagination and clinical expertise. Clinical management is rarely characterized by the administration of specific physical agents, prescriptive intervention protocols, or exclusive sets of therapeutic activities. Instead, effective intervention is often provided through eclectic and imaginative clinical approaches that consider clinical goals, patient needs, and available resources.

Attendance to the rehabilitation environment is crucial to clinical decision making and providing effective treatment and management of neurological disorders. The appropriate use of therapeutic mat tables, gait aids, simple and complex orthotics, plastic cones, therapeutic balls, biofeedback and electronic gait analysis equipment, and so on may all be integral in administering effective care. PTAs should be able to carefully survey all equipment and resources at their disposal, marry them to therapeutic goals, and then, based on the prescribed plan of care, make decisions about how to fashion a cohesive intervention regimen.

For example, say that a plan of care for a patient with a diagnosis of CVA includes gait training. A survey of clinical resources reveals the presence of mat tables, various molded ankle foot orthoses, parallel bars, canes and walkers, stopwatch and tape measures. The patient ambulates with a slow gait characterized by uneven step lengths and poor distal lower extremity control. A PTA may choose to provide a cookie-cutter-type treatment, undistinguishable from previous patient interventions. Or, a PTA may choose to fashion a customized intervention strategy. The mat table may be used for multiposition weight shifting and motor control activities, the stopwatch used to measure and monitor cadence, parallel bars and other gait devices used to fashion obstacle courses and facilitate more efficient gait, and ankle foot orthoses (with PT approval) to address knee or ankle control issues. All these activities may fit into the general category of gait training. The effective PTA sees the surrounding resources and fashions a truly customized intervention regimen to meet the patient's rehabilitation goals.

◀ Understanding Patient/Family Needs

The understanding of patient and family needs in the management of neurological disorders is critical to clinical decision making. Clinical decisions related to treatment emphasis and selection of interventions should not be made in a vacuum. The sequelae of neurological disorders significantly impact patients' functional status. Gait and other activities of daily living are necessarily affected by changes in muscle tone, hemiparesis, behavioral changes, and other common sequelae. It is important that PTAs understand a patient's or family's specific needs and expectations.

Some patients may place a greater importance on the ability to transfer to and from their bed independently. Others may place more importance on being able to perform simple kitchen duties. Some families may want their loved one to simply be as safe as possible without regard to a particular level of function. Sometimes patients are goal oriented—walking down the aisle for a child's wedding, sitting on the front pew in their house of worship, attending next year's family reunion, and so on. PTAs must take the time to discover their patients' needs. Certainly clinical decisions are heavily influenced by these needs. PTAs may decide to emphasize specific aspects of the plan of care in response to the patient's needs. PTAs may be able to foster enhanced patient compliance and cooperation by communicating the rehabilitation goals and discussing how they relate to the the patient's needs and desires.

◀ Utilization and Assessment of Objective Measures

Unlike some musculoskeletal conditions, the sequelae associated with neurological disorders can sometimes be more cumbersome to objectively measure and monitor. Guided by physical therapists, PTAs must strive to utilize the most objective measures when monitoring patient progress. The importance of objective measurement in physical therapy cannot be understated. It clearly influences, indeed drives, many clinical decisions. PTAs must be able to express patient progress (or the lack of) in more objective rather than more subjective ways. If a PTA documents that a patient's gait is improving, that statement must be supported by objective data that justifies or steers the subsequent clinical decision. If motor control is improved, the objective evidence that supports that assessment must be provided. How does a PTA know that the administered interventions are effective and his or her clinical decisions are sound? Objective comparisons to some baseline level of function or normative value help answer this question.

It is important that the most appropriate objective tool or technique be selected. Issues related to validity—the relative assurance that the tool indeed measures what it purports—and reliability—the tool's and assessor's ability to produce consistent results—must be carefully vetted. Physical therapist guidance and supervision are critical here. A wide range of measurement tools exists. Some of these tools have been carefully researched and have proven and acceptable levels of validity and reliability. Some are not as well tested and are less reliable. Some are valid and very reliable but too cumbersome to administer during routine clinical assessment. For instance, in assessing clinical progress in a patient with multiple sclerosis, a clinician may choose the following tools: Minimum Record of Disability (MRD),

MS Function Composite (MSFC), Multiple Sclerosis Quality of Life Inventory (MSQLI), Functional Assessment of Multiple Sclerosis (FAMS), or Multiple Sclerosis Impact Scale (MSIS-29) (O'Sullivan & Schmitz, 2007). The decision to use one of these assessment tools is based on reliability and validity, patient acuity, the rehabilitation setting, treatment emphasis, and other factors. Physical therapists must carefully choose assessment tools and ensure that PTAs are appropriately trained in their use (**Figure 7.3**). Appropriate training is critical to maintaining assessment reliability. PTAs should not independently choose assessment tools. If a potentially appropriate tool was not used in the initial evaluation, PTAs may discuss its use to monitor progress with the supervising physical therapist.

Gait disturbances are very common with neurological disorders. When addressing gait, PTAs must concentrate on the objective parameters

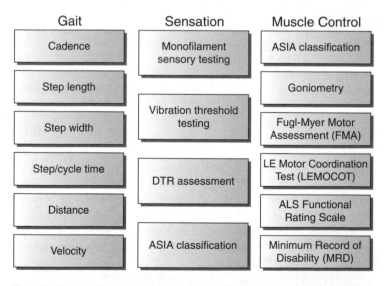

Gait	Sensation	Muscle Control
Cadence	Monofilament sensory testing	ASIA classification
Step length		Goniometry
Step width	Vibration threshold testing	Fugl-Myer Motor Assessment (FMA)
Step/cycle time		LE Motor Coordination Test (LEMOCOT)
Distance	DTR assessment	ALS Functional Rating Scale
Velocity	ASIA classification	Minimum Record of Disability (MRD)

Figure 7.3 Common Objective Measures Used in Managing Neurological Disorders

discussed previously in this text. For instance, basic observational skills combined with the use of a split-time stopwatch provide for the recording of important temporal aspects of gait. Cycle and step times are easily recorded. Cadence and left/right ratios can also be calculated and serve as a basis for the quantification of progress and gait improvement. Spatial aspects such as step/stride length and step width, though perhaps more cumbersome to measure, can also be used to quantify progress. This objective data facilitates sound clinical decision making. Decisions to alter or continue intervention strategies are better supported when quantifiable indicators of change can be applied.

Figure 7.4 shows a spreadsheet application that can be used to record and calculate objective gait parameters in a patient with CVA. Such parameters represent a more sensitive indication of change. Indeed, ambulation distance may increase without appreciable improvements in these objective parameters. Note that asymmetry in step/cycle time and stride/step length is noted and expressed as right/left ratios. If normal, these ratios would be expected to be closer to 1.0 (symmetrical). This data would certainly influence decision making. The data presented in Figure 7.4 suggest that gait is indeed improving and that the treatment strategies are likely effective. If this data were different, the PTA might make clinical decisions to alter intervention strategies. For instance, if step lengths remained constant after the first interim measurement, in an effort to produce a more efficient gait the PTA might decide to shift from ambulating in the parallel bars and concentrate more on weight-shifting and balance activities or motor control facilitation techniques.

◀ Possession of Sound Clinical Knowledge and Expertise

Sound clinical decisions can only be made if supported by a strong foundation of clinical knowledge and expertise. The components of this foundation include: (1) a clear understanding of the neurological condition, (2) an appreciation of the relationship between the sequelae and function, (3) receptivity to alternate or blended intervention strategies, and (4) the ability to fashion interventions based on the

Continuous Temporal Recordings (in seconds) (progress in %)

	Initial	Interim1	Progress	Interim2	Progress	Interim3	Progress
Date	3/3/2003	3/17/2003		3/31/2003		4/13/2003	
Right Step Time	1.86	1.35	−27%	0.92	−51%	0.86	−54%
Cycle Time	3.24	2.28	−30%	1.71	−47%	1.70	−48%
Left Step Time	1.38	0.93	−33%	0.79	−43%	0.84	−39%
Lstep/Rstep Ratio	1.35	1.45	8%	1.16	−14%	1.02	−24%
Cadence (steps/min.)	37	53	42%	70	89%	71	91%

Spatial Recordings (in centimeters) (progress in %)

	Initial	Interim1	Progress	Interim2	Progress	Interim3	Progress
Date	3/3/2003	3/17/2003		3/31/2003		4/13/2003	
Right Stride Length	62.50	72.00	15%	70.00	12%	71.00	14%
Left Stride Length	30.00	38.00	27%	52.00	73%	66.00	120%
R-L Step Length	12.00	15.00	25%	23.00	92%	32.00	167%
L-R Step Length	30.00	38.00	27%	37.00	23%	37.00	23%
R-L Step Width	15.00	15.00	0%	15.00	0%	15.00	0%
L-R Step Width	15.00	15.00	0%	15.00	0%	15.00	0%
Velocity in cm/sec.	19.29	31.58	64%	40.94	112%	41.76	117%
R/L Stride Ratio	2.08	1.89	−9%	1.35	−35%	1.08	−48%
R-L/L-R Width Ratio	1.00	1.00	0%	1.00	0%	1.00	0%
R-L/L-R Length Ratio	0.40	0.39	−1%	0.62	55%	0.86	116%

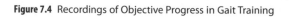

Figure 7.4 Recordings of Objective Progress in Gait Training

above foundation components. PTAs must be ever ready to receive, process, and incorporate new knowledge into their clinical arsenal. When confronted with less familiar clinical scenarios, reviewing and refreshing of concepts and facts should be the order of the day. PTAs must embrace the notion that there is always more to learn and always a means to enhance treatment efficacy, thus maintaining an inquisitive clinical demeanor.

Rather than settling into routine and unimaginative interventions, PTAs must be vigilant in providing the best customized care. For instance, say that a PTA has been assigned two patients with a diagnosis of CVA. Their outward clinical signs appear very similar. However, one patient has a medical diagnosis of middle cerebral artery syndrome and the other has a diagnosis of posterior cerebral artery syndrome. It is important that the PTA know the differences that may exist between these two syndromes (e.g., potentially more proprioceptive deficits with posterior cerebral artery syndrome). These differences may influence the types of clinical decisions and intervention strategies (Skinner & Hurley, 2007). Although the two intervention programs may be similar, the subtle clinical adjustments and decisions based on a sound knowledge of the underlying pathology may indeed provide for a more effective treatment.

Neurological conditions may fall into two broad categories: progressive and nonprogressive. For instance, CVA and traumatic spinal cord injuries are considered nonprogressive, whereas multiple sclerosis and Parkinson's are considered progressive (**Figure 7.5**). PTAs must be

Progressive Conditions	Nonprogressive Conditions
• Parkinson's • Multiple sclerosis • Amyotrophic lateral sclerosis • Alzheimer's disease • Friedreich's ataxia	• Cerebral vascular accident • Cerebral palsy • Traumatic spinal cord injury • Guillain-Barre (recovering) • Traumatic brain injury

Figure 7.5 Common Progressive and Nonprogressive Neurological Conditions

sensitive to these categories. Progressive disorders are categorized by advancing signs and symptoms. The rate of progression varies based on the condition. Clinical decisions are heavily influenced by disease type. When managing progressive disorders, in addition to providing care as prescribed by the treatment plan, PTAs must act as vigilant detectors of advancing signs and symptoms. Continuous assessment is crucial when managing progressive disorders.

When making clinical decisions, PTAs must temper their expectations of improvement with the knowledge of the progressive characteristics of the disorder. For instance, in early Parkinson's disease progression is relatively slow. Progression of symptoms in multiple sclerosis may be more unpredictable. Though the rate of progression of amyotrophic lateral sclerosis may be somewhat variable, progression of symptoms is a near certainty. It is therefore important that continuous assessment be incorporated in all management strategies.

◀ Appreciation of the Relationship Between the Sequelae and Function

Whereas recognizing, categorizing, and prioritizing sequelae is key to clinical decision making, PTAs must also be able to clearly identify the functional consequences of the sequelae. An understanding of how the sequelae impair function or task components helps drive the intervention emphasis and associated clinical decisions. Physical therapy clinicians must be proficient in performing task analysis. *Task analysis* refers to viewing whole tasks (gait, transfers, specific ADLs, etc.) and breaking them down into constituent parts (**Figure 7.6**). For instance, components for sit-to-stand transfers include anterior weight shifting, hip flexion, knee flexion, ankle dorsiflexion, quadricep control, and so on. Impairment or disability of one or more of a task's components may significantly impair function. By identifying task components and answering key questions (**Figure 7.7**) about the relationship between the sequelae and the task's components, PTAs are able to make appropriate clinical decisions related to intervention selection and modification, efficacy assessment, and goal attainment.

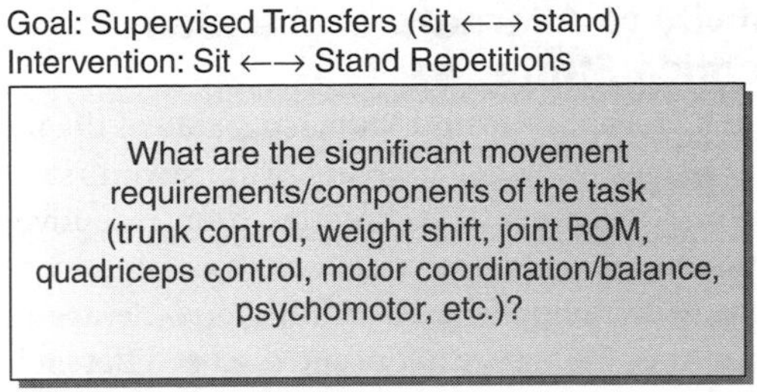

Goal: Supervised Transfers (sit ←→ stand)
Intervention: Sit ←→ Stand Repetitions
What are the significant movement requirements/components of the task (trunk control, weight shift, joint ROM, quadriceps control, motor coordination/balance, psychomotor, etc.)?

Figure 7.6 Clinical Decision-Making Task Analysis Scheme

Can the patient perform all components of the task independently or with minimal assistance?
What components cannot be performed?
What components require assistance?
What barriers exist to the performance of the task component (spasticity, rigidity, cognitive deficits, hypotonicity, apraxia, ROM loss, etc.)?
What therapeutic activities can be performed to address the barriers to performing task components?
Intervention

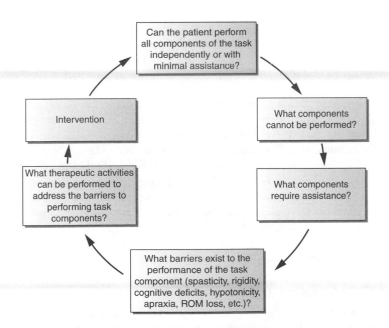

Figure 7.7 Decision-Making Query Cycle Based on Sequelae–Function Relationship

◀ Receptivity to Alternate or Blended Intervention Strategies

PTAs should be receptive to and knowledgeable of the most popular treatment strategies. Whether applying Brunnstrom's stages of motor recovery, neurodevelopmental techniques, proprioceptive neuromuscular facilitation, Frenkel's exercises, constraint-induced movement therapy, along with traditional gait, orthotic, and therapeutic interventions, PTAs must be willing to explore and discuss different intervention strategies with supervising physical therapists and hone their clinical skills (O'Sullivan & Schmitz, 2007). It is important for PTAs to understand that oftentimes academic content boundaries are blurred in the clinic. Treatment schools of thought are often blended in an effort to fashion a customized plan of care. Although clinical purists do exist, clinicians often pick and choose components of intervention strategies that best fit patient needs. For instance, treatment interventions for a patient presenting with upper extremity hypotonicity may include weight shifting onto the upper extremity (neurodevelopmental therapy), proprioceptive neuromuscular facilitation (PNF) exercise with quick stretch, the use of associated reactions to facilitate motion (Brunnstrom), and the facilitation of motion via the tonic vibratory reflex (Rood). These techniques root from disparate philosophies with varying efficacy. Clinical decisions associated with the simultaneous use of different interventions can be made only if PTAs have an understanding of the underlying rationale and efficacy of these techniques (**Figure 7.8**). When employed, this strategy must be coupled with careful assessment that guides clinical decisions to alter or continue strategies. PTAs should become comfortable with this eclectic style of treatment and participate in regular learning opportunities with supervising physical therapists and engage in continuous self-development activities.

◀ Limits on Clinical Decisions

As stated previously, physical therapy management of neurological disorders is often characterized by complex plans of care with multiple goals. In making sound clinical decisions, PTAs should carefully

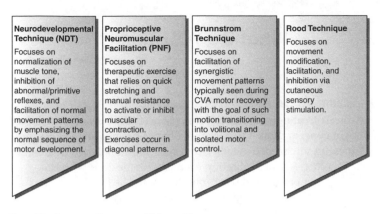

Figure 7.8 Common Treatment Philosophies

prioritize these goals, relate them to varied sequelae, and implement clinical interventions consistent with the prescribed plan of care. PTAs may have great latitude in clinical decisions related to intervention selection. However, there are limits on those clinical decisions. PTAs must implement intervention strategies that address all prescribed goals. Prioritizing goals does not mean ignoring goals. PTAs may not ignore goals or portions of the prescribed treatment plan. Selected interventions must be inclusive and representative of the entire prescribed plan of care.

◀ References

O'Sullivan, S. B., & Schmitz, T. J. (2007). *Physical Rehabilitation* (5th ed.). Philadelphia, PA: F.A. Davis.

Skinner, S. B., & Hurley, C. (2007). *Pocket Notes for the Physical Therapist Assistant.* Sudbury, MA: Jones and Bartlett Publishers.

What Do YOU Think?

▶ **Scenario 1 (Level I)**

You are treating a patient who suffered a left CVA resulting in flaccid right upper and lower extremities. The treatment plan includes therapeutic exercise, bed mobility, transfers, and ambulation training.

1. What type of facilitation exercises can be done with this patient today and what muscles should be facilitated first?
2. As this patient begins to get muscle return, how might this patient benefit from PNF?

▶ **Scenario 2 (Level II)**

You are treating a patient who has suffered a traumatic brain injury and is experiencing balance problems with ambulation. The treatment plan calls for static and dynamic balance training. List three dynamic balance exercises you could do with this patient. How can you assess the patient's progress with these exercises?

Level I Activity

▶ **Physical Therapy Evaluation**
Patient Name: _____

HPI: Pt. is a 75-year-old female s/p right CVA two weeks ago resulting in left hemiparesis and expressive aphasia. Pt. was admitted to an inpatient rehabilitation facility yesterday. Pt. is being seen for PT, OT, and speech therapy.

PMH: HTN, IDDM

MEDS: Aldomet, diabeta

SH: Pt. lives with her husband in an apartment with five steps to enter. Stairs have a railing on the right side. Prior to admission, pt. was independent in ADLs.

Mental Status: Unable to fully assess mental status secondary to pt.'s expressive aphasia. Pt. is able to follow commands without difficulty.

ROM: Right UE and LE and left LE are WNL throughout. Pt. displays no active movement of the left UE. Passively the left UE is WNL.

Muscle Strength: Right UE and LE are Normal throughout. Pt. displays zero strength throughout left UE. Pt. displays left hip flex. F, hip abd. F+, hip ext. F+, knee ext. F+ and knee flex F+ and ankle DF/PF F-.

Sensation: Pt. has decreased sensation to light touch on the left UE and LE.

Pain: Pt. without complaints of pain.

Muscle Tone: Pt. displays no abnormal muscle tone.

Balance: Sitting—pt. is able to sit unsupported. Standing—pt. is able to stand with minimal assist.

Functional Status: Pt. is able to roll to the right with moderate assist and to the left with supervision. Pt. transfers supine ←→ sit with mod. assist, sit ←→ stand with mod. assist. Pt. ambulates with wide base quad cane for 20 feet with min. assist for occasional loss of balance. Pt. ambulates with a steppage gait.

Problems: Decreased active movement, decreased strength, decreased balance, dependency in functional skills.

Short-Term Goals: Pt.'s left hip flex, abd. and ext. strength will increase a half a grade. Pt.'s left knee strength will increase a half a grade. Pt. will roll independently. Pt. will transfer supine ←→ sit ←→ stand with min. assist. Pt. will ambulate with a wide base quad cane for 60 feet with min. assist for balance.

Long-Term Goals: Pt. will be independent in transfers. Pt. will ambulate with an appropriate assist device with supervision for 100 feet.

Assessment: Pt. is motivated and very cooperative. Pt. appears to be a good rehab. candidate.

Plan: Daily PT for therapeutic exercise, balance training, bed mobility, transfers, and ambulation training.

Instructions: The physical therapist completed this evaluation yesterday and has asked you to treat this patient today. After completing the treatment write a progress note and answer the following questions.

1. What ambulation training did you give this patient today and why?
2. What treatment was given to address this patient's gait deviations?
3. What balance activities could be done to improve this patient's gait?

Level II Activity

▶ **Physical Therapy Evaluation**
Patient Name: _____

HPI: Pt. is a 55-year-old female who was involved in a motor vehicle accident and sustained a traumatic brain injury. Pt. suffers from double-vision, muscle weakness, and changes in mental status since the accident. Pt. was admitted to inpatient rehabilitation yesterday. Pt. is being seen for PT, OT, and speech therapy.

PMH: None

MEDS: Dilantin

SH: Pt. lives with her husband and children in a home with two flights of steps. Stairs have a railing on the right side. Prior to admission pt. was independent in ADLs and ambulation.

Mental Status: Pt. is alert and oriented ×3 but often makes inappropriate comments.

ROM: Bil. UE and LE PROM is WNL throughout.

Muscle Strength: Left UE shoulder F+, elbow and wrist F; left LE hip flex. F, abd. P+, IR/ER F, ext. P; bil. knee flex/ext F+ and bil. ankle DF P and PF F. Unable to assess muscle strength secondary to abnormal muscle tone.

Sensation: Intact in response to light touch throughout.

Pain: Pt. has no complaints of pain.

Muscle Tone: Pt. displays moderate spasticity in her right upper and lower extremity. Pt. displays a flexor synergy in her UE and an extensor synergy in her LE.

Balance: Sitting balance—able to sit unsupported. Standing—requires mod. assist to maintain static standing balance.

Functional Status: Pt. is able to perform all bed mobility with min. assist. Pt. transfers supine ←→ sit with min. assist, w/c ←→ bed with mod. assist. Pt. amb. the length of the parallel bars with mod. assist. to assist with weight shifting and balance.

Problems: Decreased strength, decreased balance, and dependency in functional skills.

Short-Term Goals: Pt.'s strength will increase a half a grade in her UE and LEs. Pt. will perform bed mobility with CG. Pt. will transfer supine ←→ sit with CG and w/c ←→ bed with min. assist. Pt. will be able to stand unsupported with CG. Pt. will amb. with appropriate device for 50 feet with CG.

Long-Term Goals: Pt. will be independent in bed mobility and transfers. Pt. will be independent with an appropriate assistive device on level surfaces and stairs.

Assessment: Pt. is cooperative and appears to be a good rehab. candidate.

Plan: Daily PT for therapeutic exercise, balance training, bed mobility, and transfers and ambulation training.

Instructions: The physical therapist completed the evaluation yesterday and has asked you to treat this patient today. After completing the treatment write a progress note and answer the following questions.

1. What type of therapeutic exercise can be done to address the patient's spasticity?
2. Identify two standing-balance exercises that can be done with this patient.

Clinical Decision Making in Administering Therapeutic Exercise

When executing an exercise regimen, PTAs must rely on sound knowledge and expertise. Sound knowledge of the functional significance of muscular anatomy and kinesiology is essential. A fine appreciation of synergistic relationships, reversal of muscle actions, passive/active insufficiency, and other concepts clearly influences therapeutic exercise selection and modification.

Therapeutic exercise is the backbone of physical therapy intervention. Most physical therapy patients will ultimately require some type of exercise during their treatment course. Therapeutic exercise is an integral part of the overall plan of care. Modalities, transfer/ambulation training, and other physical therapy interventions in isolation are rarely effective. When most people think of exercise, strength training comes to mind. However, therapeutic exercises include flexibility, coordination, and balance activities as well as strengthening exercises. Additionally, therapeutic exercises may be initiated to increase range of motion, improve endurance, and enhance cardiopulmonary function.

In many cases, the PT therapeutic exercise plan is less, rather than more, prescriptive. Physical therapists assume that based on the objective data and treatment goals outlined in the initial evaluation, competent PTAs can make effective clinical decisions in choosing appropriate therapeutic exercise interventions. Competent PTAs use their knowledge of anatomy, pathology, kinesiology and other clinical sciences when making therapeutic exercise decisions. Clearly, in instances of selected orthopedic surgery rehabilitation, strict and quite prescriptive exercise and rehabilitation protocols may be in place. Absent such protocols, PTAs must guard against a rote and unimaginative selection of exercise regimens. Therapeutic exercise clinical decisions are influenced by the diagnosis, goals, behavior of symptoms, patient needs, long-term goals, and so on. Once specific exercise techniques have been selected, PTAs must also make clinical decisions related to number of repetitions and other therapeutic exercise variables.

◀ Goals of Treatment

In order to select the correct exercise regimen, PTAs must understand patient problems and the goals set toward correcting those problems. Other than the most common goals, such as improving range of motion and strength, therapeutic exercise is most useful in enhancing balance, improving cardiopulmonary function, and increasing endurance (**Figure 8.1**). By carefully cataloging the deficits outlined in the initial evaluation and drawing on a sound knowledge of anatomy, competent PTAs select exercises that target the appropriate muscles, joints, and/or functions.

The skill of carefully reading and understanding the clinical significance of the initial evaluation cannot be understated. Oftentimes therapeutic exercise goals are implicit rather than explicit. For instance, a plan of care for a patient recovering from a hip fracture may include "therapeutic exercise." One likely intervention goal is to achieve

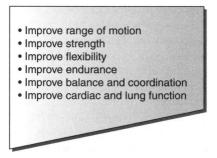

- Improve range of motion
- Improve strength
- Improve flexibility
- Improve endurance
- Improve balance and coordination
- Improve cardiac and lung function

Figure 8.1 Common Goals of Therapeutic Exercise

independence in transferring sit to stand. Competent PTAs recognize that difficulty in transfers may be related to a combination of muscle weakness in the upper or lower extremities. The patient may have difficulty pushing up using the upper extremities, necessitating exercise emphasis on triceps strengthening. Perhaps the patient is having difficulty extending the knee while weight bearing, necessitating more emphasis on quadriceps strengthening. PTAs must be able to recognize underlying patient problems and translate them into exercises that become part of the exercise program.

PTAs must prioritize patient problems and goals. For example, a patient may have a severely tight gastrocnemius as well as a weak tibialis anterior. The goals for this patient may be to improve strength and range of motion at the ankle. However, which goal should be addressed first? In this case, drawing on sound knowledge of kinesiology, competent PTAs would likely make the clinical decision to initially concentrate on gastrocnemius lengthening before being able to effectively strengthen the antagonist muscle group.

Besides prioritizing patient problems, PTAs need to be sure that the chosen exercises enable the patient to meet prescribed goals. To make these decisions, PTAs must understand the concepts of therapeutic exercise. For example, to improve endurance the muscle is worked at a submaximal level, which is usually safe to perform even in the early stages of recovery (Kisner & Colby, 2007). Plans of care may not necessarily spell out the number of repetitions the patient is to perform on any given day. It is up to the PTA to look at a goal involving endurance and make the clinical decision to decrease the amount of resistance and increase the number of repetitions, as appropriate. PTAs must be able to link each exercise performed to a treatment goal. The PTA needs to constantly reassess the patient's progress and problems to ensure that the exercise program allows the patient to reach his or her full potential.

◀ Attendance to the Rehabilitation Environment

It is important that PTAs make optimal use of clinical space and equipment. Therapeutic equipment varies from facility to facility. Once clinical decisions regarding the appropriate type of exercise have been made, the next decision to make is how that exercise will be completed. For instance, when addressing severe weakness the use of manual or gravity-only resistance may be indicated. When addressing mild-to-moderate weakness, cuff weights, dumbbells, and elastic resistives may be more appropriate. However, once again, physical therapists do not typically provide a prescriptive therapeutic exercise plan that specifies each activity, number of repetitions, and so on. These are significant and critical clinical decisions that competent PTAs must make.

PTAs must not only recognize what exercise is appropriate, but also be able to select the most effective equipment. In some instances, there may be no difference between using dumbbells or cuff weights. Other times, dumbbells may be preferred if the cuff weights cannot be securely fastened. Still other times, elastic resistives may be more appropriate because of the particular exercise, line of pull of the muscle, or the amount of muscle strength.

Some facilities have a wide variety of therapeutic exercise equipment—treadmills, stationary bikes, upper body ergometers, standalone joint-specific isotonic units, variable resistance and isokinetic units, and so on. Although these machines are all effective, PTAs must select the most appropriate equipment. PTAs can easily slip into bad habits of throwing a patient on a machine just to keep the patient "busy" while they are treating someone else. Can machines be used to assist with time-management issues? Yes, as long as the machine is selected with the patients' rehabilitation goals in mind and there is sound rationale for using the device. When PTAs place a patient on a machine they should ask: "Why is the patient being placed on the machine?" For example, if a treadmill is being used as a warm-up device, then the patient may be placed on the treadmill for 5 to 10 minutes at a slow speed. In contrast, a patient who needs the treadmill for endurance training or strengthening would require a different protocol.

To ensure therapeutic effectiveness and patient safety, PTAs should be comfortable with all available equipment so they can make informed clinical decisions when carrying out the therapeutic exercise plan. In facilities where there is not a lot of equipment available, clinicians need to use their sound knowledge of anatomy and kinesiology and their creativity to design effective exercise programs. Competent PTAs attend to their environment by not only using their space and equipment effectively, but also by facilitating compliance by making exercise more enjoyable—or at least interesting—for patients. This may include transforming therapeutic exercise activities into games or functional activities, such as weighted-ball throwing/kicking or functional activities that mimic activities of daily living.

◀ Understanding Patient Needs

When implementing an exercise program, PTAs need to be aware of precautions or patient limitations. Patients' needs are related to myriad factors, including age, diagnosis, overall fitness, premorbid condition, and personal and rehabilitation goals. For example, a patient recovering from a coronary artery bypass graft surgery (CABG) would benefit from lower extremity active range of motion exercise, whereas resistive and upper extremity exercises would likely be inappropriate. PTAs must also understand all postsurgical precautions as they relate to prohibited motions (e.g., post total hip replacements) and alter exercises accordingly. PTAs must monitor patients' responses to exercise. For instance, they must be able to recognize and understand the signs of and responses to fatigue and the significance of muscle soreness following exercise and be able to alter the exercise program accordingly. Of course, all patients are different, and even those with the same diagnosis may tolerate exercise differently.

Exercise programs need to carry over to functional activities. PTAs need to understand the specific needs of their patients in reference to their everyday life. A clear understanding of what the patient hopes to achieve in therapy or the difficulties the patient is having at home allows the PTA to better customize the exercise program. Whenever exercise can include patients' interests or activities they enjoy, patients become more motivated and treatments become more effective. For example, if a patient with a traumatic brain injury (TBI) loves soccer, a PTA may decide to address coordination and balance deficits by having the patient maneuver a soccer ball through an obstacle course of cones. Although treadmills offer patients the ability to ambulate long distances on a smooth surfaces, the outside world is not always perfectly smooth. A PTA needs to recognize the patient's reality with respect to the outside world and know when it is time to transition a patient from a treadmill to an obstacle course with uneven surfaces.

PTAs use information about patients' past medical history, lifestyle, and life stage to make decisions as to the type of exercise or exercise position. For instance, PTAs may choose to limit position changes—supine to prone to standing and then back to supine—for patients with moderate to severe arthritis. Not only would such multiple position changes likely be painful for the patient, but it would also increase the time needed for the treatment. Although exercises using a therapeutic ball are effective for trunk stabilization activities, an elderly patient might not feel comfortable sitting on a ball. It is up to the PTA to consider these issues and make appropriate decisions to optimize the therapeutic exercise program.

◀ Utilization and Assessment of Objective Measures

PTAs need to constantly reassess the effectiveness of patients' exercise programs. PTAs use formal and informal assessments. PTAs use visual observations as well as quantitative measurements to assess progress or lack of progress. For example, if a patient has difficulty performing 10 repetitions of knee extension on Monday and on Wednesday the patient is able to easily complete 10 repetitions of the same exercise, satisfactory progress in gaining muscle strength may be assumed. The PTA must not only recognize this progress but also change the patient's exercise regimen accordingly. The first clinical decision to be made is to determine that the exercise program needs to be changed. The next decision to be made is how. The PTA has the choice to increase the number of repetitions, add resistance, change the exercise position, or change the type of exercise (i.e., open chain to closed chain or from isotonic to isokinetic). Once again, this decision should be based on the treatment goals and individual patient needs. No matter what decisions are made, all observations, interventions, changes, and reasons for treatment should always be documented.

Besides observation, PTAs have other tools to measure progress, including manual muscle testing (MMT) and goniometry. Both goniometry and MMT are accepted quantitative measurement procedures and, depending on the diagnosis and treatment goals, are routinely performed. In some instances, isokinetic testing may be used to objectively assess parameters of muscle strength. Although this testing is usually ordered by the physical therapist on a routine schedule, PTAs may be called upon to assist in completing such testing. Oftentimes, PTAs are not specifically told when to assess patient progress. However, effective PTAs recognize changes in patients' status and make the clinical decision to measure and document changes—or lack of changes—as appropriate. Whether therapeutic exercise is being used to enhance balance, improve strength, increase endurance and cardiopulmonary status, decrease gait deviations, and so on, PTAs must strive to provide valid and reliable objective evidence of efficacy and progress.

◖ Possession of Sound Clinical Knowledge and Expertise

When executing an exercise regimen, PTAs must rely on sound knowledge and expertise. Sound knowledge of the functional significance of muscular anatomy and kinesiology is essential. A fine appreciation of synergistic relationships, reversal of muscle actions, passive/active insufficiency, and other concepts clearly influences therapeutic exercise selection and modification. With a sound knowledge of the muscular system, clinicians have a better understanding of how to exercise specific muscles and muscle groups more effectively. PTAs must also rely on sound knowledge of basic exercise concepts. For instance, PTAs should understand the relationship among intensity, duration, and frequency (Kisner & Colby, 2007). For example, if a patient is receiving daily physical therapy, a PTA may decide to decrease the intensity and/or the duration of the treatment so as not to fatigue the patient (**Figure 8.2**). A patient with moderate arthritis

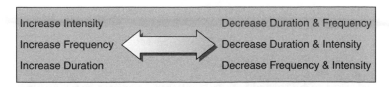

Increase Intensity	Decrease Duration & Frequency
Increase Frequency	Decrease Duration & Intensity
Increase Duration	Decrease Frequency & Intensity

Figure 8.2 Therapeutic Relationship Among Intensity, Duration, and Frequency

may benefit from isometric rather than isotonic exercise. A patient with a shoulder complex disorder may benefit from performing exercises in the supine position to better stabilize the scapula.

The physical therapist's initial evaluation provides PTAs with patient problems and treatment goals. Once PTAs have a good understanding of these issues, they must begin to make a number of clinical decisions. The first decision to be made is what type of exercise the patient needs. Is the problem a lack of range of motion requiring stretching, or weakness requiring strengthening exercises, or a balance deficiency requiring static and dynamic exercises?

If the patient needs stretching, the PTA must make a clinical decision as to the type of stretch (self vs. passive stretch), position and repetitions, and when within the treatment session the stretch should be performed. Once again, these decisions are influenced by the loss severity, patient needs, goals, competing disorders, and so on. The PTA must use his or her sound knowledge of muscles and length–tension relationships as well as the extent of the deficit and the patient's needs to determine the best possible stretch activity. For example, if the patient has severe tightness of the gluteus maximus, the patient may be placed in quadruped position and asked to rock posteriorly. However, if this same patient has decreased balance, knee pain, or is elderly, the quadruped position may not be appropriate. Instead, the PTA may make the clinical decision to place the patient in supine position and provide passive knee-to-chest exercise. By the same token, if the patient has complaints of stiffness or pain at the hip, the PTA may make the clinical decision to administer the knee-to-chest exercise at the beginning of the treatment session to assist in increasing ROM and to warm up the hip.

If a patient needs strengthening exercises, PTAs have even more clinical decisions to make. Based on sound knowledge of MMT and pathology, PTAs need to determine the type of strengthening exercise appropriate for the patient—isotonic, isometric, or isokinetic. This decision is made with sound knowledge of diagnosis along with an understanding of the current recovery phase—acute, subacute, or chronic—and treatment goals. Two patients with the exact same muscle strength may need to be treated with two different exercises based on their diagnosis. One patient may tolerate minimal resistive isotonic exercise, while the other—due to pain with movement—may better benefit from multi-angle isometric exercise. All too often, clinicians get in a habit of using one type of exercise (usually isotonic exercise) and forget the benefits of isometric and isokinetic exercise (Kisner & Colby, 2007). **Figure 8.3** provides summary definitions of these types of exercise.

Once the clinical decision of what type of strengthening is made, the decision-making process continues. For example, if isotonic exercise is selected, would the patient benefit from open-chain versus closed-chain exercise? Again, this decision is based on sound knowledge and understanding of the patient's diagnosis and stage of healing. PTAs need to not only understand the difference between open-chain and closed-chain activities, but also know the importance of both. It is not uncommon to observe PTAs instructing lower extremity exercise in sitting, prone, and supine positions, but less often in the standing position. Closed-chain activities provide opportunity for muscles to contract in a more functional fashion and therefore may play an important role in returning the patient to premorbid activities.

PTAs must also consider the strength of the muscle when choosing specific exercises. PTAs and physical therapists are considered experts in MMT and must use their skills to select exercises that

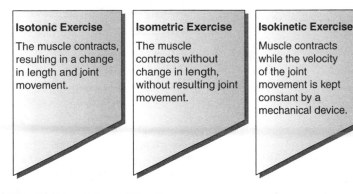

Isotonic Exercise

The muscle contracts, resulting in a change in length and joint movement.

Isometric Exercise

The muscle contracts without change in length, without resulting joint movement.

Isokinetic Exercise

Muscle contracts while the velocity of the joint movement is kept constant by a mechanical device.

Figure 8.3 Common Types of Exercise

challenge the muscle. PTAs must be able to use the MMT results and translate the information into an effective exercise regimen. Through sound knowledge, PTAs select the motion, position, type of muscular activity—concentric or eccentric—and level of resistance or assistance (**Figure 8.4**).

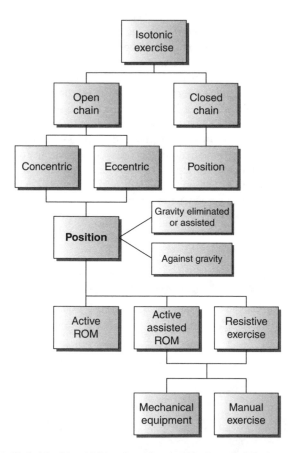

Figure 8.4 Clinical Decision-Making Considerations for Isotonic Exercise

Novice PTAs sometimes appear to more randomly determine the amount of resistance for a particular isotonic exercise. For example, say that a 65-year-old female is assigned to a PTA for strengthening of hip musculature following a fall. The PTA instructs the patient in straight leg raises with a 5-pound cuff weight at the distal leg. How did the PTA determine that 5 pounds was the appropriate resistance? Should the determination of resistance be an arbitrary clinical decision? Resistance is a crucial dosage parameter in isotonic resistive exercise. It should be carefully considered, monitored, and altered. The Daily Adjustable Progressive Resistive Exercise (DAPRE) program and the Delorme and Oxford techniques represent systematic means of determining resistance dosage and progressive resistance during the treatment session (Hall & Thein Brody, 2005). **Table 8.1** summarizes these dosage and progression techniques. Whichever technique is chosen, effective PTAs ensure that appropriate resistance is provided and progression is systematic.

After all these decisions are made, the PTA finally selects an exercise. One exercise may not work for all patients. Depending on a number of variables—pain, mood, edema, and so on—the same exercise that was effective for a patient on Monday may not be appropriate on Wednesday. Effective PTAs develop a repertoire of diverse exercise activities to accomplish therapeutic goals. Such diversity should include a variety of exercise types. For example, isometric exercise

Table 8.1 Isotonic and Resistive Exercise Dosage and Progression Regimens

Technique	Initial Dosage Determination Based on Maximum Number of Repetitions (RM)	Progression During Session
Delorme	10 rep maximum	1 set at 50%, 10 RM 1 set at 75%, 10 RM 1 set at 10 RM
Oxford	10 rep maximum	1 set at 10 RM 1 set at 75%, 10 RM 1 set at 50%, 10 RM
DAPRE	6 rep maximum	1 set at 50%, 6 RM 1 set at 75%, 6 RM As many reps as possible at 6 RM and adjust for next day

activities should not be neglected. Muscle-setting exercises are often used with patients in the early stages of healing, but as a patient progresses multiple-angle isometrics and stabilization activities may be used to improve strengthening, postural stability, and dynamic stabilization (**Figure 8.5**).

Isokinetic exercise allows the patient to receive resistance throughout the range of motion (**Figure 8.6**). Patients exercise against the force of the maximum dynamometer speed. Although offering resistance throughout the range of joint motion can be very beneficial, it is not appropriate for every patient. Although isokinetic exercise is usually specifically ordered within a plan of care, PTAs can suggest the idea to the physical therapist when appropriate. Of course, the real question is when it is appropriate. Effective PTAs develop sound rationales for a new intervention prior to making the suggestion. Isokinetic machines are often used toward the end of the rehabilitation process or with patients who are pain free and are able to produce enough force to

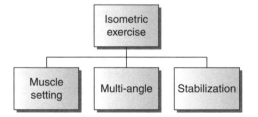

Figure 8.5 Clinical Decision-Making Considerations for Isometric Exercise

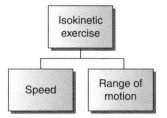

Figure 8.6 Clinical Decision-Making Considerations for Isokinetic Exercise

push against the machine. It should be noted that typically, no matter who first thought of implementing isokinetic exercise, the physical therapist provides the PTA with the specific isokinetic regimen.

Strengthening exercise possibilities are infinite. The key is to use sound knowledge and understanding of the theories behind the different forms of exercise in combination with knowledge of specific exercises and, of course, imagination to formulate an effective exercise program. The determination of dosage and repetitions during traditional progressive resistive exercise was discussed previously. However, effective PTAs understand and may also manipulate the relationship between body position and resistance placement to alter muscular load.

When performing straight leg raises, the placement of a 10-pound cuff weight proximal to the knee rather than at the distal leg—thereby greatly reducing the resistance arm—alters the resistance effect of the weight (**Figure 8.7**). Placing a patient in the prone position and performing shoulder flexion activities from the mid-range to the end range—altering the affect of gravity and required torque production—requires increased muscular demand at the end range as opposed to performing the exercise while sitting. Here again, such clinical decisions must be based on a sound foundation of academic

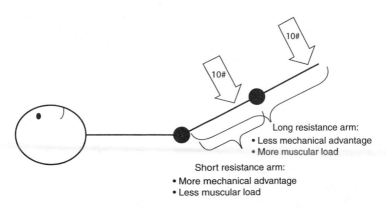

Figure 8.7 Alteration of Muscle Load Through Manipulation of the Resistance Arm

and clinical knowledge. These clinical decisions must be individualized for each patient, related to functional needs, and focused on goal attainment.

As mentioned earlier, PTAs must also understand the concepts of fatigue, muscle soreness, and specificity of training. A patient's current pathology, past medical history, mental status, age, and current physical condition impact exercise choices. And once a great exercise has been selected, if the patient does not like it, has difficulty performing it, or is not comfortable doing the exercise, the process begins again. When the patient finally performs the selected exercises, the PTA must comprehend the impact of the exercise and then use sound knowledge to determine what happens next. PTAs must not only recognize when particular exercises are not working—for whatever reason— they must also be able to use problem-solving skills backed by a sound knowledge base to make adjustments.

◀ Thinking Outside the Box

Once the problems and goals of exercise are understood and decisions about the type of exercise have been made, the specific exercise is selected. When selecting exercises, PTAs must use sound knowledge and their imagination. An exercise can usually be performed in more than one way. An innovative PTA not only uses sound knowledge but refrains from doing the same exercises with each patient. Innovative or diverse exercise activities do not have to be earth shattering or groundbreaking, but may be more fun for the patient. For example, if a patient needs an open-chain quadriceps strengthening exercise against gravity, the PTA has a number of options. The patient can sit in a chair and perform full arc knee extensions or the patient can sit in a chair and perform full arc knee extensions, kicking a small ball every time the knee is extended.

Sometimes creativity with exercise does not come from the PTA's imagination but rather from sound clinical knowledge of activities or exercises that are used less often and are sometimes forgotten. Two examples of this are the use of PNF (Proprioceptive Neuromuscular Facilitation) and plyometrics. All too often, PTAs have a bag of exercises that they use every day. If, however, PTAs dig into their memories, they will recover many unused resources or therapeutic concepts that can be used to accomplish treatment goals.

PNF is often used with patients with neurological problems (e.g., CVA, TBI, etc.). PNF uses diagonal patterns to facilitate movement in a more functional manner while stimulating proprioceptors (Voss, 1985). But what about patients with orthopedic problems or patients with general deconditioning? Can these patients also benefit from PNF? A PTA may consider the benefits of PNF as well as other treatment considerations and make the clinical decision as to how beneficial PNF would be for a particular patient (Skinner & Hurley, 2007). **Figures 8.8** and **8.9** summarize the therapeutic benefits and treatment considerations for PNF.

Plyometrics are another example of strengthening exercises that are not routinely used, and certainly not with all types of patients. However, plyometrics can be very effective in improving power and coordination at the end of the rehabilitation process. Of course, plyometrics may not be appropriate for every patient. The clinician must

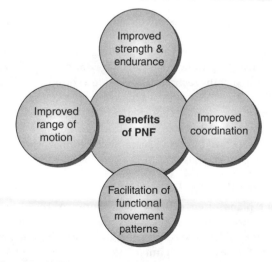

Figure 8.8 Benefits of PNF

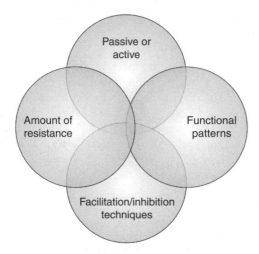

Figure 8.9 Treatment Considerations for PNF

consider a patient's age, past medical history, strength, balance, and coordination.

Once all the clinical decisions regarding exercise have been made, PTAs must use their knowledge and understanding of modalities and other physical therapy techniques to create a sound overall treatment regimen. The placement of the exercise regimen at a specific point in the treatment is a decision that should be based on an overall sound clinical knowledge base. Once again, PTAs need to have a sound rationale for all aspects of the plan of care. Such rationale should be linked to achieving patient goals.

◖ Limits on Clinical Decisions

Treatment plans often call for therapeutic exercise, progressive resistive exercise (PRE), or just upper and lower extremity exercise. In these cases, PTAs are responsible for most decisions regarding the design of the exercise regimen. In some instances, PTAs are limited in their decision making because of postoperative protocols.

Sometimes the physical therapists provide quite prescriptive exercise regimens. In these instances, PTAs must be diligent in determining what constitutes management of the prescribed plan and what activities or changes require formal PT consultation and assent.

◀ References

Hall, C. M., & Thein Brody, L. (2005). *Therapeutic Exercise: Moving Toward Function* (2nd ed.). Philadelphia, PA: Lippincott Williams & Wilkins.

Kisner, C., & Colby, L. A. (2007). *Therapeutic Exercise: Foundations and Techniques* (5th ed.). Philadelphia, PA: F.A. Davis.

Skinner, S., & Hurley, C. (2007). *Pocket Notes for the Physical Therapist Assistant.* Sudbury, MA: Jones and Bartlett Publishers.

Voss, D., Ionta, M., & Myers, B. (1985). *Proprioceptive Neuromuscular Facilitation: Patterns and Techniques* (3rd ed.). Philadelphia, PA: Harper & Row.

What Do YOU Think?

▶ **Scenario 1 (Level I)**

The patient is a 67-year-old female with a diagnosis of osteoarthritis of the right knee resulting in mild knee pain. Patient's right knee range of motion is within normal limits. Patient's muscle strength is fair-plus at the knee. The treatment plan calls for therapeutic exercise for strengthening, and the short-term goal is to increase knee strength to good so that the patient can ambulate on stairs without difficulty.

1. Describe three exercises, in detail, that may help this patient achieve her goal. Offer your rationale for each exercise
2. For each exercise that you described, name the muscle(s) that is being strengthened.

▶ **Scenario 2 (Level II)**

The patient is a 25-year-old male recovering from a right meniscectomy that was performed two weeks ago. The patient's range of motion is right knee flex/ext −10 to 110 degrees. The patient's right knee strength is fair-minus for quadriceps and poor-plus for hamstrings. The treatment plan calls for stretching and strengthening exercises for the right knee.

1. Select one self-stretch and one passive stretch for this patient. Include the name of the muscle stretched in each.
2. Select four strengthening exercises for this patient. Offer your rationale for each exercise.

▶ **Comparing Scenarios 1 and 2**

1. Although the treatment plans for the patients in Scenarios 1 and 2 are similar, discuss why each patient should be approached differently.
2. Discuss other considerations that need to be contemplated when treating each patient.

Level I Activity

▶ **Physical Therapy Evaluation**

Patient Name: _____

Diagnosis: Adhesive capsulitis, left shoulder

History: Patient is a 53-year-old male who presents with a chief complaint of left shoulder pain and stiffness. The patient states that he has had increased symptoms in the last two weeks following raking leaves outside. The patient apparently saw his doctor in January. Therapy was recommended. However, patient began to feel better and did not follow up on physician's suggestion. Patient states that the pain is "not as bad" as it was in January.

Patient states that he had surgery on left shoulder 15 years ago for "removal of tumors" and an "old football injury." He began having intermittent pain two years ago following continuous overhead activities. Patient states that the pain is "not bad" now, but he notes that it has begun to worsen. He describes the pain as a "tightness with activities" with occasional morning "numbness" of the left arm. Pain is 5/10 in the left shoulder with overhead activities.

Objective Finding: Inspection reveals no major asymmetries. Palpation is negative for pain or abnormality. Range of motion at the left shoulder reveals 120 degrees of abduction, 140 degrees of flexion, 20 degrees of external rotation, and normal internal rotation. Patient has pain at the end ranges of all movements. End feel for all movements is capsular. Strength of the left shoulder is generally graded as 3.5–4/5 and 5/5 on the right.

Resisted movements do not reproduce pain. Cervical nerve root strength tests are negative for weakness. Cervical range of motion is within normal limits. Deep tendon reflexes are present and equal bilaterally.

Assessment: Patient presents with signs and symptoms consistent with an adhesive capsulitis, as evidenced by a capsular pattern of tightness at the left shoulder. Some weakness of the left shoulder muscles is also noted. The patient would benefit from physical therapy for restoration of normal shoulder range of motion and strengthening activities.

Goals: STG: ROM of the left shoulder will increase 10 degrees, pain will decrease to 3–4/10 on pain scale.

LTG: Left shoulder ROM will be WNL, strength of left shoulder will be 4+/5.

Plan: Physical therapy two times a week for moist heat/cold packs, passive stretching, and therapeutic exercise.

Instructions: Patient was evaluated by the physical therapist at his last visit. Perform a treatment on this patient, write a progress note, and then complete the following questions.
  1. Which exercises would you perform and why?
  2. What effect may the modalities have on the exercises?

Level II Activity

▶ **Physical Therapy Evaluation**
  Patient Name: _____

Diagnosis: Right knee injury

History: The patient is a 15-year-old male who injured his knee two months ago. The patient states that he was "playing around" in his room and fell onto his right knee. He states that he had no immediate pain. About 5 minutes following the injury he felt "something rubbing together" in his knee. He had pain with flexion and pain during the night. The next morning there was edema and stiffness and pain with ambulation. X-rays were negative for fracture. The patient currently complains of pain on "the inside of my knee" and pain with weight bearing and shifting.

Objective Findings: The patient is 6' 4". Palpation of the right knee reveals tenderness over the tibial pole of the right medial collateral ligament and the medial underside of the patella. The patient states that the medial pain started approximately two weeks ago. Anterior draw test on the left is positive for laxity. No collateral laxity noted. McMurray's test is negative. Quadriceps strength is left 5/5 and right 4–/5 and hamstring strength is right 5/5 and left 4–/5. Inspection reveals minimal edema right knee. Range of motion is WNL bilaterally.

Assessment: Patient presents with symptoms consistent with a possible grade I sprain of the right medial collateral ligament of the knee. He also presents with symptoms consistent with possible cartilage damage at the patellofemoral joint. The patient also has some laxity of the left anterior cruciate ligament. The patient would benefit from physical therapy for pain management and strengthening activities.

Goals: STG: Increase strength one-half grade for quads and hamstrings.

LTG: Increase knee strength to 5/5.

Plan: Suggest physical therapy twice weekly for three to six weeks. Physical therapy to include quad strengthening on the right, hamstring strengthening on the left, and moist heat/ice.

Instructions: The patient was evaluated at his last visit. Perform a treatment on this patient, write a progress note, and then complete the following questions.

1. Provide the rationale for each exercise you selected for this patient.
2. The patient leaves your facility and goes home and develops increased pain. When he returns to your facility two days later, the patient states that he has had increased pain since his last treatment. What do you do?

Level II Activity

Refer to the scenario from the previous activity. Three weeks have passed, and the patient is no longer experiencing pain. The patient states that he is getting bored with his exercises and asks if there are any other things he could be doing. He also states that he would like to go back to playing basketball as soon as possible.

Instructions: Perform another treatment on this patient using this revised information and then complete the following questions. Keep in mind that there have been no changes in the treatment plan.

1. What changes did you make to the treatment and why?
2. What activities can be done with this patient to assist him in achieving his goal of being able to play basketball?

Clinical Decision Making in the Provision of Pediatric Physical Therapy Services

Patients with neurological disorders tend to require complex intervention strategies. The multiple sequelae associated with central nervous system disorders combined with the associated affects on motor development make the provision of physical therapy to pediatric populations quite challenging. It may take a PTA several years to become truly proficient in providing physical therapy to children with neurodevelopmental disorders.

Physical therapist assistant participation in pediatric treatment varies based on geography, state regulation, and the clinical setting. Pediatric physical therapy is often complex and atypical. Children are not little adults. Treatment of children requires patience, innovation, and a keen awareness of developmental, psychological, physical, and social differences as compared to adults. PTAs involved in pediatric care work best when teamed with a physical therapist pediatric specialist. Pediatric physical therapy treatment plans are often less—rather than more—prescriptive. Typically, treatment plans do not outline exactly how to accomplish each goal. Like adults, children—even those who are the same age and who have the same diagnosis—may present with differences that affect response to treatment. Effective PTAs must place a very high premium on using interventions that accomplish the treatment goals and keep the child engaged.

❖ Goals of Treatment

Most pediatric patients fall into two broad categories: those with long-term neuromuscular problems and those with acute orthopedic or deconditioning problems (**Figure 9.1**). Treatment goals vary greatly depending on the patient category. For instance, if the patient has an orthopedic problem or is deconditioned, the plan of care usually includes therapeutic exercise and functional activities. Such plans are similar to those of adults, minus those modalities that are contraindicated with children. Treatment goals are also similar to those of adults. Goals may include decreasing pain, increasing range of motion, gaining muscle strength, and improving functional activities. Effective PTAs make clinical decisions on how to accomplish these goals using age-appropriate activities, oftentimes only limited by their imagination. For example, although a short-arc quad set may improve quadriceps strength in a

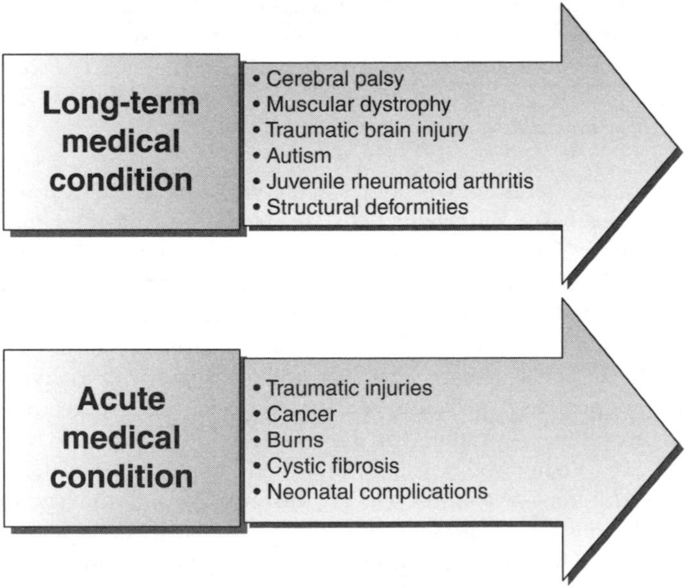

Long-term medical condition
- Cerebral palsy
- Muscular dystrophy
- Traumatic brain injury
- Autism
- Juvenile rheumatoid arthritis
- Structural deformities

Acute medical condition
- Traumatic injuries
- Cancer
- Burns
- Cystic fibrosis
- Neonatal complications

Figure 9.1 Common Pediatric Problems

teenager, it will take a little more work to convince a four-year-old to perform the same exercise.

Patients with neurological disorders tend to require complex intervention strategies. The multiple sequelae associated with central nervous system disorders combined with the associated affects on motor development make the provision of physical therapy to pediatric populations quite challenging. It may take a PTA several years to become truly proficient in providing physical therapy to children with neurodevelopmental disorders. Physical therapist plans of care often call for the use of neurodevelopmental techniques (NDT) or other motor control strategies that enhance functional abilities. Such techniques are often only a small part of entry-level PTA education. PTAs hone their skills through close association and mentoring from physical therapist pediatric specialists, practical experience, and participation in formal continuing education.

Goals may be stated in functional terms, outlining major developmental milestones. PTAs must convert the goals and treatment plan into specific techniques, which may include altering postural reflexes and normalizing muscle tone. PTAs must be able to choose specific techniques needed to accomplish patient goals. For example, a patient with cerebral palsy who has moderate-to-severe extensor tone may have a goal to sit independently. The patient's muscle tone needs to be controlled in order to accomplish the goal of sitting. With a plan of care that includes NDT and motor control activities, the PTA must select appropriate activities to decrease muscle tone in order to accomplish the goal of sitting.

◀ Attendance to the Rehabilitation Environment

The treatment of children occurs in a variety of environments, including acute care hospitals, inpatient rehabilitation facilities, school settings, outpatient facilities, and the home. Patient diagnoses vary widely from setting to setting. PTAs must attend to the rehabilitation environment when planning their daily treatment, because the environment significantly influences what activities can be performed. In acute care hospitals, patients are medically unstable and therapy is usually done at the bedside or in a PT gym on a limited basis. Much attention must be paid to patients' medical conditions. Patients may be ambulated in the hallways and assisted with transfers out of bed into chairs. In this case, exercise equipment and space is limited to what can be in patients' rooms.

In inpatient rehabilitation hospitals, patients are usually more medically stable and need intensive rehabilitation and continued medical attention. In this setting, clinicians have more time to spend with patients compared to acute care hospital settings. Patients usually receive one-on-one therapy to optimize functional ability. Equipment typically is plentiful and includes pediatric gait aids, modified pedal cycles, specially designed toys, therapeutic balls, and so on. Effective PTAs creatively match existing equipment with therapeutic goals.

School settings vary depending on the type of school. In schools for children with disabilities, sensory and motor equipment will be plentiful. When making clinical decisions about physical therapy activities, PTAs will have a wide variety of equipment to choose from, including toys that have been adapted to children with disabilities common to that environment. Of course, space and equipment must be shared in a busy therapy gym. At times, PTAs may decide to work with other therapists and patients to perform specific activities (e.g., kicking a ball or basketball activities). At other times, especially if a child has problems attending to tasks, PTAs may need to make the clinical decision to treat their patient in a quiet secluded area.

In school settings, goals and interventions must pertain to or impact the school environment. Physical therapy must address the child's needs within the classroom. When making clinical decisions, PTAs must consider all equipment available as well as other issues in the classroom. For instance, a PTA may decide to use the school's recreational playground equipment in therapy sessions. Effective PTAs also work with the classroom teacher to try to provide continuity to goal attainment. For example, if the child's goal is to climb up and down stairs reciprocally, the PTA needs to involve the classroom teacher in this goal so that each time the patient goes to gym or to art class he or she is provided cues on proper stair climbing. In all pediatric settings—but especially in school settings—the PTA must be an active member of the interdisciplinary team. Effective PTAs cannot make clinical decisions in a vacuum. Communication and agreement among members of the interdisciplinary team—teacher, occupational therapist, speech therapist, and so on—are crucial.

In public school settings, PTAs may need to pay more attention to their environment. Public schools do not always have the facilities and equipment that schools for children with disabilities do. Often, only a limited number of students in a particular school may receive therapy. Most public schools do not have a PT gym, and therapy is performed in empty classrooms or hallways. PTAs must attend to their environment to make clinical decisions on how to use their environment to its optimal potential. PTAs must use their knowledge of the patient's goals and plan of care, scan the surrounding environment, catalog assets and drawbacks, and then make decisions as to how best to proceed. For example, in the absence of balance equipment, a PTA may decide to put tape along the floor in the hallway and have the patient perform tandem walking along the line. A PTA may decide to take a child out to the playground and use a hopscotch game as a balance and coordination activity. Effective PTAs work very closely with the physical therapist pediatric specialist in identifying and initiating appropriate therapeutic strategies.

Attendance to the environment also pertains to home care settings. At times, patients with acute medical, chronic, and developmental conditions receive home care for varying periods of time. Effective PTAs attend to the environment around them and use the patient's home to its full potential. This might include incorporating the child's favorite toys into the intervention session. PTAs should think outside the box, or maybe just outside the house, and use the backyard or courtyard to perform ball activities and endurance training. When the outside environment is not appropriate, PTAs need to ask parents for a cleared space to work without distractions from the TV or family members. However, sometimes it is effective to incorporate siblings or other family members into parts of the treatment regimen.

Besides being attentive to their actual physical environment, PTAs need to also attend to the different levels of supervision in the different clinical settings. PTAs must understand and adhere to the supervision requirements as specified by state regulations. In some states, supervision in certain pediatric settings—especially those treating patients with chronic conditions—requires contact with the physical therapist via telephone communication only. PTAs must be able to make clinical decisions within the plan of care and must keep the lines of communication open and know when communication with the PT is needed. Once again, however, optimal care is best facilitated when the PTA is closely teamed with the physical therapist pediatric specialist.

◀ Understanding Patient Needs

Patient needs vary by population. A child's needs in an acute care facility are necessarily much different from those in a school setting for children with long-term disabilities. For instance, a child in an acute care hospital being treated for an orthopedic condition may be scared being in a strange place and afraid of anyone who walks through the door in a white coat. This patient needs to understand exactly what physical therapy will entail in the most simple of terms. The patient may also be in pain, and the thought of ambulation on non–weight-bearing crutches may seem impossible. PTAs must not only understand these feelings but expect them. If patient reactions are anticipated, clinicians can plan ahead.

For example, an eight-year-old patient with a long leg cast requiring non–weight-bearing ambulation training may present significant challenges. Such challenges may include emotional immaturity, poor motor capabilities, an inability to fully understand instructions, and so on. A PTA may make the decision to initially see the patient with one or two parents in the room to assist with explanations, keep the patient calm, and explore training and functional options. If the treatment is done at the bedside, the PTA needs to bring all equipment in at one time so that the PTA can remain with the patient throughout the session. When dealing with children, PTAs must place a premium on fun and entertainment—the language of childhood. As stated earlier, children are not small adults. Even in dire situations PTAs must remain sensitive to children's general psyche and consider ways to make the therapy entertaining.

When treating children with significant medical conditions, such as cancer, PTAs need to consider the patient's medical status during treatment. Even very young children are able to express feelings of fatigue and pain. Clinicians must be attentive to a variety of cues—both verbal and nonverbal—and adjust intervention strategy accordingly.

Children with long-term disabilities have other needs. Most children with physical disabilities receive physical therapy for years. Although some children also have mental disabilities, not all do. PTAs must consider the patient's mental capacity in order to provide effective treatment. Children with mental disabilities may require simple commands. They may need to be redirected during intervention sessions. Remember that in the school setting PTs and PTAs are active members of the interdisciplinary team. Physical therapy intervention may incorporate behavior modification or other social concerns identified by other professionals. When working with difficult cases, effective PTAs look to the other members of the team to gain insight and direction.

Some children with physical disabilities do not have mental limitations and should not be treated as if they do. Many of these children have been through extensive therapy with a number of therapists and know their limitations and abilities better than the clinicians. PTAs need to interact with these patients on an age-appropriate level. Patients need to know that the clinician understands them. PTAs must strive not to make therapy "boring." PTAs need to understand that the more challenging the therapy, the more fun it needs to be. Children, like adults, tend to want to stay within their comfort zone. Effective physical therapy often pushes patients out of the comfort zone. When therapy is disguised in a creative activity, the child may not mind being pushed to the limits.

When a child is beginning treatment with a new PTA, the child needs to feel comfortable with the clinician. Despite great efforts to reassure patients, some young children are very attached to their parents. During the initial visits, PTAs may decide to allow the parents in the treatment area and then slowly wean the child away from them. PTAs can use creativity to facilitate the separation process. For example, a PTA might suggest that the parent needs to make a phone call, speak with a nurse, or run out to the store—something to get the parent out of the room. Ultimately, the child will feel more comfortable and be able to separate from his or her parent. Separating the child from the parent allows for less distractions and more directed treatment.

PTAs must not only consider the needs of the patient, but also the needs of the parents. Parents want the best for their children. Many parents are very involved in the recovery or treatment of their children.

PTAs need to understand that parents need to be involved. Whether parents are eager to get involved or a bit hesitant, parent participation is crucial. It is important for parents to reinforce the work the child is doing in therapy. Further, effective PTAs are careful in how they communicate with parents. Parents often present with a range of psychological coping mechanisms related to the child's condition. Whether denial—"After a few months of therapy, I know my child will catch up"—or depression—"My child has no chance of having a normal life"—effective PTAs must be attentive to parent coping mechanisms and take care to appropriately communicate with parents. If a PTA notes that a parent is having a difficult time coping with a child's disability, the PTA should consult the supervising physical therapist for interaction advice and appropriate intervention.

Parents must be an integral part of the management team. They need to understand the goals and objectives of therapeutic activities. They also need to understand the crucial role they play in their child's treatment. PTAs need to be able to give parents clear directions on exercises and activities for children to continue during nontherapy time. Effective PTAs are sensitive in how they integrate parents into therapeutic activities. Parents must be parents—not surrogate clinicians. Whenever possible, parental therapeutic activities should be incorporated into functional activities such as dressing and feeding. Effective PTAs spend time training parents on how they can best participate in reaching the child's goals. Clinicians need to be realistic and consider parents' time constraints, other siblings, and available resources. At times, PTAs must be conscious of the need for supportive services and discuss those needs with the supervising physical therapist. Parents may need support accepting realistic goals for their children. PTAs can support parents by assisting the patients to achieve their highest potential while at the same time emphasizing the children's abilities.

◖ Utilization and Assessment of Objective Measures

What assessment tools are used depends on the child's age, mental status, and pathology. PTs perform evaluations on children with acute medical conditions using tools similar to those used with adults, with some adjustments made for age, neurological development, and pathological condition. PTAs need to use objective measurements to periodically assess patients' progress toward goals and treatment effectiveness.

A number of pediatric assessment tools are available for patients with neurological problems (**Figure 9.2**). Some tools emphasize motor function, whereas others emphasize sensory perception, proprioception, muscle tone, or reflexes. If the child is in the school setting, testing results and goals will become part of the child's Individual Education Program (IEP) or Individual Family Support Plan (**Figure 9.3**).

- Movement Assessment in Infants
- Alberta Infant Motor Scale
- Denver Developmental Screening Test
- Peabody Developmental Motor Scales
- Bruininks-Oseretsky Test of Motor Performance
- Purdue Perceptual Motor Survey

Figure 9.2 Common Pediatric Assessment Tools
Source: Ratliffe, (1998), p. 56.

Individual Education Program (IEP)	Individual Family Support Plan (IFSP)
Plan used for school-age children to guide educational staff and related service providers through the year, including an outline of services to be provided, short- and long-term goals, and reassessment periods (Ratliffe, 1998, p. 125).	Plan used for children under the age of three. Includes plan of services to be provided, goals and objectives, as well as family needs (Ratliffe, 1998, p. 7).

Figure 9.3 An IEP Versus an IFSP

PTAs must understand the tool(s) that the therapist selects so that they can fully comprehend the results of the test and related goals. PTAs should use portions of the tool to intermittently assess progress. For example, if a portion of a measurement tool assesses how long a child can perform single-leg stance, the PTA should periodically assess single-leg stance during treatment. Formal reassessment will be performed by the PT, but it is important that PTAs assess the patient's progress toward IEP goals. No matter the age of the patient or the tools used, it is important to use objective data to monitor patient progress.

◖ Possession of Sound Clinical Knowledge and Expertise

When treating pediatric patients, PTAs must rely on sound clinical knowledge to make clinical decisions in selecting the most appropriate activities. When it comes to children with acute medical conditions, PTAs must have a good understanding of the pathological condition and medical treatment. Clinicians must then be able to anticipate how the pathology will impact functional skills. Sound knowledge of precautions and contraindications enables clinicians to make educated decisions as to types of exercise and activities to choose. PTAs must understand that normal vital sign ranges for children are different from those for adults.

Many of the clinical decisions that are made for children are similar to those made for adults. However, PTAs must be able to adapt therapeutic activities to the patient's age. Finally, PTAs must understand the patient's prognosis, because it may influence their clinical decisions. For example if a PTA is performing gait training with a child with a debilitating disease and a poor prognosis, the clinician may choose to use a walker rather than crutches with the rationale that the walker will provide more stability to a patient who is getting weaker.

When treating pediatric patients with neurological problems, PTAs must, first and foremost, understand the patient's initial evaluation. Clinicians must be familiar with the evaluation tool the physical therapist selected and be able to comprehend the results. PTAs must also have sound clinical knowledge of normal development as well as knowledge of tonic and postural reflexes and effects of abnormal tone. It is only through understanding normal development that clinicians can fully assess, recognize, and alter abnormal development. PTAs must have sound knowledge and understanding of therapeutic exercise, including stretching and strengthening and balance and equilibrium exercises, as well as know how to best facilitate or inhibit muscle tone.

Once the PTA is able to observe abnormal movement or function, the clinical decisions begin. Effective PTAs recognize the sources of abnormal movement patterns. For example, if a child is observed to have asymmetries in gait, a number of questions arise: Where are the asymmetries coming from? Does the child have fluctuating tone? Does the child have a muscle imbalance? Does the child have a leg-length discrepancy? What impact do the asymmetries have on function? Is the child tripping or falling? How will the asymmetries affect higher level skills, such as running, jumping, or hopping? These are only some of the questions that clinicians must ask themselves. Clearly, these questions will be answered in the physical therapist's evaluation. However, effective PTAs have a heightened sensitivity to these questions and read the PT evaluation with a critical eye, looking to immediately translate objective findings into functional consequences.

Once these initial questions are answered, PTAs must decide what activities can be done with this child in order to reach the established goals. PTAs must be able to implement a variety of activities to accomplish a single goal. Remember, depending on the child's age, the patient's attention span may be limited or he or she might simply not like the toy or activity that was selected. Effective PTAs are ready with multiple backup strategies. Age and cognitive capacity will also impact which activities will be appropriate for the patient. For example, two children ages five and seven with normal cognitive function will like different activities. Of course, one of the simplest things to do is to ask the child his or her likes and use those activities in a therapeutic fashion. For example, consider the four-year-boy who loves puzzles and needs to work on trunk stabilization and balance in half-kneel. The clinician can take out a stack of puzzles, put the patient in half-kneel position, and allow him to complete puzzles on a coffee table.

PTAs should continuously ask themselves whether the activities they have selected are helping to meet the patient's goals. Clinicians need to understand how to provide effective treatment while at the same time keeping the child engaged. PTAs who have a sound foundation of pediatric pathologies and normal development and good observation skills will be able to use their imagination to accomplish their patients' goals in a fun environment.

◀ Limits on Clinical Decisions

Plans of care for pediatric patients with acute medical problems may be quite specific with regards to precautions, contraindications, and standardized protocols. Plans for patients with long-term neurological problems tend to be less prescriptive. With more complex patients, the PT might not delegate all aspects of the plan to the PTA. PTA clinical decision making may therefore be limited by the delegated portion of the plan. Effective PTAs only make clinical decisions they are most comfortable with. The importance of effective and open communication with the supervising PT is critical.

◀ References

Dreeben, O. (2007). *Introduction to Physical Therapy for Physical Therapist Assistants.* Sudbury, MA: Jones and Bartlett Publishers.

Effgen, S. K. (2005). *Meeting the Physical Therapy Needs of Children.* Philadelphia, PA: F.A. Davis.

Ratliffe, K. T. (1998). *Clinical Pediatric Physical Therapy: A Guide for the Physical Therapy Team.* St. Louis, MO: Mosby.

What Do YOU Think?

▶ **Scenario 1 (Level I)**

Patient is a 13-year-old girl with a diagnosis of leukemia receiving medical treatment in an acute care hospital. Patient's range of motion is within normal limits throughout. Patient's muscle strength is fair minus in both lower extremities and fair in both upper extremities. The patient is independent in transfers and ambulation but displays decreased endurance. The treatment plan calls for therapeutic exercise for strengthening, and the short-term goal is to increase lower extremity strength to fair plus and improve endurance so that patient can ambulate 300 feet without rest.

1. Describe three exercises, in detail, that could help this patient achieve her goal. Provide a rationale for each exercise.
2. Discuss how the patient's age and diagnosis influence her treatment.

▶ **Scenario 2 (Level II)**

Patient is a 10-year-old girl with a diagnosis of mild athetoid cerebral palsy. Patient is able to transfer and ambulate independently but is unable to perform unilateral stance or hop or skip. The treatment plan calls for balance training.

1. Describe three age-appropriate activities that could be used to improve the patient's balance.
2. Based on the information presented, what other functional skills might be impacted by the patient's poor balance?

▶ **Scenario 3 (Level II)**

Patient is a five-year-old boy with a diagnosis of spastic cerebral palsy. Patient rolls independently but is not able to maintain prone on elbows. Patient is able to sit independently but is unable to stand. Patient is able to maintain static sitting for short periods of time.

1. Describe two activities that promote prone on elbows.
2. How could a therapeutic ball be used with this patient?

Level II Activity

▶ **Physical Therapy Evaluation**

Patient is an eight-year-old girl who was developing normally until the age of four, when she sustained a TBI resulting in right hemiplegia.

PMH: TBI

MEDS: None

SH: Pt. lives with parents. Child wears a right AFO daily.

Mental Status: Unable to fully assess mental status secondary to pt.'s expressive aphasia. Pt. is able to follow commands without difficulty.

ROM: Left UE and LE are WNL throughout. Right UE AROM flex 0–120, abd 0–90, IR/ER 0 degrees, elbow flex/ext 0 degrees, wrist flex 60 degrees, ext –60 degrees.

Right LE hip	PROM	AROM
Flex	WNL	WNL
Abd	30°	25°
Ext	5°	0°
Knee flex	WNL	WNL
Ext	0°	–5°
Ankle		
DF	5°	0°
PF	10°	0°

Muscle Strength: Left UE and LE are normal throughout. Right UE shoulder flex and abd 3+, IR/ER 1, elbow flex/ext 0, wrist flex 1, ext 0.

Sensation: Intact in response to light touch.

Pain: Patient has no complaints of pain.

Muscle Tone: Positive hypertonicity in right UE > right LE.

Balance: Standing balance poor; unable to SLS or tandem walk. Poor coordination secondary to decreased AROM on right side.

Functional Status: Patient transfers and ambulates independently. Asymmetrical gait pattern noted. Maintains right LE in ER and displays decreased heel strike.

Other Observations: Maintains right UE in flexor synergy.

Problems: Decreased active movement, decreased strength, decreased balance, dependency in functional skills.

Short-Term Goals: Increase strength to 4+/5 on right LE. Increase endurance—pt. will ambulate on treadmill ×10 min. Independent in-home exercise program.

Long-Term Goals: Pt. will be independent in school activities.

Assessment: Pt. is motivated and very cooperative. Pt. appears to be a good rehabilitation candidate.

Plan: PT 2×/wk for therapeutic exercise, balance training, and endurance training.

Activity: This patient was evaluated at her last visit. Based on the information provided, perform a treatment on this patient and write a progress note. Answer the following questions.
   1. Provide the rationale for each exercise you selected for this patient.
   2. Design a home exercise program for this patient.

Level II Activity

▶ **Physical Therapy Evaluation**
Patient is a five-year-old boy with a diagnosis of developmental delay and seizure disorder. The child suffered a TBI at age three. Child has mild hearing loss.

ROM: Bilateral upper extremity and lower extremity are within normal limits.

Strength: Specific manual muscle test not performed due to patient's age, but gross assessments for all extremities are within normal limits.

Tone: Patient displays increased extensor tone in bilateral lower extremities in supine position.

Reflexes: Patient displays integrated reactions for the following reflexes: flexor withdrawal; extensor thrust; ATNR, STNR; tonic labyrinthine prone and supine; righting reactions; and landau. Patient displays good protective reactions in sitting. Patient displays equilibrium reactions of abduction and shoulder flexion but tends to fix lower extremities.

Functional Observation: Patient displays good head control.

Prone: Patient is able to maintain prone on extended arms with good head control and is able to weight shift and reach for objects.

Supine: Patient displays an increase in tone in bilateral lower extremities. Patient does not like this position and tends to push himself up with his upper extremities to get into sitting.

Rolling: Patient rolls using his upper extremities to push himself over, with his lower extremities following with good dissociation between trunk and pelvis.

Sitting: Patient sits independently in ring position or long sitting with a posterior pelvic tilt.

Crawling: Patient is able to crawl independently with dissociation and a wide base of support but is not used functionally.

Kneeling/Standing: Patient kneels independently. Patient is not able to stand through half kneeling. Instead, patient tends to bear crawl into standing or pull up on furniture. Patient ambulates independently with bilateral shoulder retraction and elevation, arms in a high guard position, increased lumbar lordosis and bilateral hip abduction and internal rotation. Increased plantar flexion is noted with increased speed. Patient is not able ambulate up and down stairs reciprocally.

Assessment: Patient is a five-year-old boy with a diagnosis of developmental delay who has problems with equilibrium, ambulation, and stair climbing.

Goals: Patient will be able to get in and out of sitting position independently. Patient will assume standing through half kneel four out of five times. Patient will be able to ambulate with increased speed with decreased plantar flexion. Patient will be able to climb up and down five steps with one handrail with supervision four out of five times.

Treatment Plan: Physical therapy 3×/week for therapeutic exercise and balance and ambulation training.

Activity: This patient was evaluated at his last visit. Perform a treatment and write a progress note. Answer the following questions.
1. Provide the rationale for each exercise you selected for this patient.
2. Design a home exercise program for this patient.

Clinical Decision Making in the Provision of Geriatric Physical Therapy Services

Geriatric patients have different needs than other patient populations. Many have unique psychological and social needs. In addition, some geriatric patients have extensive secondary medical problems that influence rehabilitation effectiveness. The psychological and cognitive changes that older patients might experience may require PTAs to alter their teaching strategies.

People aged 60 years and older comprise the fastest growing segment of the U.S. population. Medical advances and improvement in general health status (nutrition, fitness, etc.) have increased life expectancy. The so-called "elderly" are increasingly living healthy, active lives and must frequently mesh their lifestyle with limiting physiological phenomena associated with aging. The geriatric patient may be treated in various physical therapy settings. From a 70-year-old with lateral epicondylitis to an 82-year-old amputee, physical therapy clinicians must be sensitive to the particular needs and physiological changes associated with aging. Physical therapy clinicians must also be aware of the psychosocial issues and implications associated with aging. Effective PTAs are not only competent in providing physical therapy to geriatric patients, they also understand the needs and special circumstances of older adults.

◀ Goals of Treatment

Physical therapy for geriatric patients includes promoting optimal health and function. The PT will set specific goals based on the patient's problems and diagnoses. However, these goals are often tempered by the patient's age and lifestyle. For example, when treating a relatively sedentary geriatric patient with hip pain, a therapist may set a goal to restore the patient's range of motion to within functional limits as opposed to within normal limits. Because of anatomical and physiological changes, it may be unrealistic to restore the patient's complete range of motion. However, this does not mean that the patient cannot have functional motion that allows for the performance of all or most activities of daily living. As PTAs make clinical decisions about therapeutic activities, they must be sensitive to preexisting conditions that may influence the types of goals the PT ascribes to therapy.

PTAs must be aware of how the therapeutic goals relate to the patient's lifestyle and living conditions. Does the patient live alone? Is the patient a community ambulatory? Does the patient need to regularly negotiate steps? The answers to such questions are important in effectively implementing a physical therapy regimen to improve gait. If the patient lives in a home with two flights, it is important to emphasize stair climbing, safety, and endurance during gait training. However, if a patient is returning to a nursing home, although the general goal may be the same, the treatment emphasis may be very different.

Given the normal physiological changes associated with aging, including loss of muscle mass, decreased cardiorespiratory endurance, and so on (**Figure 10.1**), geriatric patients have a higher risk of falling (Dreeben, 2007;

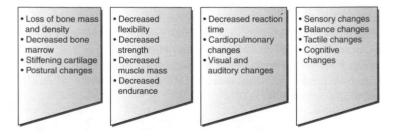

• Loss of bone mass and density • Decreased bone marrow • Stiffening cartilage • Postural changes	• Decreased flexibility • Decreased strength • Decreased muscle mass • Decreased endurance	• Decreased reaction time • Cardiopulmonary changes • Visual and auditory changes	• Sensory changes • Balance changes • Tactile changes • Cognitive changes

Figure 10.1 Age-Related Changes in the Geriatric Population

Pagliarulo, 2007). In many instances, physical therapy goals specifically target fall prevention. PTAs must understand the risk factors associated with falls and adjust their actions accordingly. PTAs must be sensitive to contributing factors such as poor eyesight or minor equilibrium impairment that may impact the selection of therapeutic activities.

Effective PTAs ensure that patients are able to easily draw the connection between the physical therapy goals and individual needs and personal goals. PTAs discuss the goals with their patients. Clearly, being attuned to the patient's needs is a universal requirement for effective physical therapy. However, sometimes with older adults the personal goals may be related to an upcoming event. For instance, a patient may be most concerned about walking down the aisle at a grandchild's wedding, negotiating the ramp of a cruise ship, or getting into and out of a bathtub independently. Armed with the knowledge of patient's personal goals, PTAs can more effectively fashion a treatment regimen consistent with the overall plan of care and therapeutic goals.

◀ Attendance to the Environment

PTAs will encounter geriatric patients in a number of settings. Treatment, expectations, and the types of required clinical decisions may differ based on the rehabilitation environment. Whether using a large font when synthesizing a home exercise program or using step stools to help patients negotiate treatment tables, PTAs must carefully attend to the rehabilitation environment and ensure that they can address the special needs of the geriatric population.

As stated earlier, the overall improvement in the general health status of the elderly has positively impacted longevity and quality of life. It is not unusual for physical therapy clinicians to treat otherwise healthy geriatric patients with orthopedic disorders more typically associated with a younger patient population. More frequently, these patients are being seen side-by-side with younger patients with sport- or recreation-related injuries and disorders.

Of course, geriatric patients are still seen in great numbers in acute care and rehabilitation facilities. In an acute care hospital, patients—at least initially—tend to be medically unstable. If the patient is medically unstable, PTAs must consider the precautions and contraindications that must be adhered to based on the patient's diagnosis. PTAs must be aware of the limitations and benefits of providing physical therapy at the bedside or in the department gym. Once the patient is medically stable, clinicians need to assist in preparing the patient for discharge. PTAs may need to make the clinical decision to call in the physical therapist to adjust goals and change the plan of care. With time, goals may change from prevention of further disability to promotion of functional activities.

While other healthcare workers are developing a discharge plan, PTAs need to progress the patients as efficiently as possible, focusing on functional activities. In order to accomplish this goal PTAs must know what equipment is available. If a patient is being discharged to another facility, that facility will review the patient's medical record, looking for the progress the patient is making. If the patient is being discharged home, the PTA may need to adjust therapeutic interventions while staying within the scope of the plan of care. For example, if the plan calls for transfer and ambulation training and the patient has 18 steps to enter his home, the PTA needs to make ambulation on the stairs a priority during each session. In this case, rather than using practice stairs that are typically found in a rehabilitation gym, it may be more important to practice stair climbing on a real staircase to better approximate home conditions.

Geriatric patients may also be seen in subacute settings, short-term rehabilitation hospitals, skilled nursing facilities, and extended care facilities. The goals and treatments in each facility may differ, but ultimately the objective is to make the patient as functional as possible. The amount of time the clinician has to treat the patient may also differ depending on the facility. PTAs need to be able to work within the constraints of the facility while at the same time prioritize different aspects of treatment.

Geriatric patients also receive home care. Depending on state regulations, PTAs may treat patients at home under the supervision of a physical therapist. PTAs need to be aware of possible dangers or obstacles in the home. Through discussions with the family and information from the physical therapist, PTAs may make the clinical decision to focus on specific problems as they relate to ADLs. Due to the limited availability of equipment in the patient's home, PTAs must be creative. Clinicians are not able to carry all of their equipment with them, so they must assess the home and determine ways to use household objects therapeutically. For example, a PTA may decide to have the patient hold on to the kitchen counter while performing hip flexion, abduction, and extension exercises in the standing position.

Geriatric patients are often seen in outpatient clinics for various physical therapy problems. Although equipment in outpatient facilities tends to be abundant, not all equipment may be appropriate for use with geriatric patients. Clinicians may need to exercise caution in taking patients on and off equipment—especially those patients who have limited mobility and/or balance impairments. Some geriatric patients treated in outpatient facilities have already received physical therapy in a hospital, rehabilitation facility, or at home and are coming to the outpatient facility to continue intervention. Other patients will be coming to the outpatient facility for management of minor injuries or problems. When making clinical decisions, PTAs must understand where the patient is in the rehabilitation process in the context of the therapeutic goals.

◀ Understanding Patient Needs

Geriatric patients have different needs than other patient populations. Many have unique psychological and social needs. In addition, some geriatric patients have extensive secondary medical problems that influence rehabilitation effectiveness. The psychological and cognitive changes that older patients might experience may require PTAs to alter their teaching strategies. For example, instructing the older patient in the use of new assistive devices and alteration of gait patterns may require additional practice and cueing. PTAs may need to make clinical decisions based on the patient's cognitive abilities and comfort level. For example, a geriatric patient who has been ambulating with a walker for a period of time and is physically ready to progress to a cane may be hesitant. The patient may feel safer with the walker. The PTA may need to spend additional time explaining the benefits of progression to a cane. The PTA should not disregard the idea of advancing the patient to a cane, but the progression may need to proceed more slowly than usual.

Many geriatric patients are experiencing social changes, such as those associated with retirement, loss of a spouse, or loss of independence. PTAs need to understand that these major changes can impact rehabilitation. Social changes may impact the patient psychologically and decrease motivation during the rehabilitation process. PTAs may need to find ways to enhance motivation. In some instances, attending regular physical therapy sessions can become a social outlet for an elderly patient living alone. In such cases, the PTA may make the decision—in preparation for discharge—to speak to the PT about possible referral to adult day care or other community programs.

PTAs must also understand how the patient's needs may be impacted by his or her past medical history and other secondary medical problems. For example, a patient may have been admitted to the hospital with an ankle fracture resulting in a short leg cast necessitating non–weight-bearing ambulation. Let's say that this patient also has a past medical history of two recent myocardial infarctions. To ambulate safely, the patient may need multiple rest periods, and the PTA must closely monitor the patient's vital signs.

Because of the social, physical, cognitive, and psychological changes associated with aging, PTAs often must make clinical decisions not based solely on a patient's primary diagnosis. Instead, PTAs must consider the whole patient. The goal of providing the most effective and safe physical therapy remains primary. Effective PTAs must be aware of the special needs of this population and tailor rehabilitation interventions appropriately.

◄ Utilization and Assessment of Objective Measures

As with all patients, PTAs must continuously assess the geriatric patient's progress. Although many of the assessment tools used in the general younger adult population are also used with geriatric patients, some tools are used primarily with the older population. For example, manual muscle tests, goniometry measurements, and sensory tests are used for all patient populations. However, balance tests, mental status or psychological assessments, and fall prevention screenings tend to be used more often with geriatric patients.

Clinicians must understand all tests and screenings and understand how their results influence therapeutic goals. PTAs should understand how the tests are administered. This understanding may provide opportunity for the incorporation of testlike activities in the therapeutic regimen. If the formal assessment includes a battery of tests, the PTA may be able to make the decision to select one test from the battery to assess treatment efficacy between formal reassessments.

In other instances, PTAs may make decisions regarding treatment ideas based on the results of the tests. For example, if a patient displayed a high risk of falling, a PTA may decide to treat the patient in the physical therapy gym as opposed to the bedside or to set up the therapeutic environment to mimic "at-risk" home conditions.

PTAs must always use objective measures to determine patient progress toward therapeutic goals. Objective measurement techniques must be safe and easily administered. Because these measurement techniques vary—especially those related to balance and fall risk—PTAs must work very closely with PTs in determining the best measures. Note that the goals synthesized by the PT will always be influenced by the patient's overall condition and needs. PTAs should caution against being guided by established norms that may not take into account patient variability. PTAs must carefully document objective progress and use such data to alter the treatment within the plan of care to facilitate goal achievement.

◀ Possession of Sound Clinical Knowledge and Expertise

Clinicians must consider a number of issues when treating geriatric patients. PTAs must understand normal age-related changes, specific pathologies common to geriatric populations, and psychosocial issues that occur with older adults.

A number of "normal" age-related changes occur as people get older. These changes affect different systems in the body and need to be considered when treating geriatric patients (Figure 10.1). PTAs must be able to alter treatment within the scope of the plan of care to accommodate these age-related changes. PTAs must also be able to recognize normal age-related changes versus those related to a particular medical diagnosis. For example, when performing gait-training activities with geriatric patients, PTAs must consider that older adults naturally display decreased trunk rotation, decreased step length, and decreased speed and that none of these limitations may be related to the patient's diagnosis. PTAs must be sensitive to the fact that aging and age-related physiological changes are not pathological; they are a normal aspect of physiological progression. It is crucial for PTAs to discern the differences between pathology and aging and apply therapeutic concepts accordingly.

When treating geriatric patients, PTAs must know the common pathologies seen in this population. These common pathologies may be documented as part of the patient's past medical history or history of present illness. PTAs must understand the impact these pathologies have on the patients' rehabilitation and make clinical decisions accordingly. For example, if the patient has a past medical history of arthritis, the PTA needs to understand what type of arthritis the patient has and which joint(s) are affected. The PTA then considers the limitations that the arthritis may cause, such as decreased motion, edema, joint deformity, pain, and functional limitations. Next, the PTA must determine the possible effects of these limitations on physical therapy. For instance, will the patient's functional activities be impacted by the patient's arthritis? Will the pain interfere with progress toward the patient's goals? Will the patient's arthritis have an influence when selecting an assistive device and gait pattern?

Acute medical problems may also be complicated by common pathologies such as infection, pneumonia, congestive heart failure, or a previous cerebral vascular accident. PTAs need to use their knowledge of these pathologies when making clinical decisions. For example, a patient who is admitted with a hip fracture and then suffers from a myocardial infarction or has congestive heart failure is most likely going to progress more slowly and will require more modification of the rehabilitation than a patient without such complications. Besides progressing more slowly, the PTA should recognize the need to take cardiac precautions and closely monitor the patient's vital signs.

Patients may also suffer from decubiti, contractures, muscle atrophy, and deconditioning while in the hospital secondary to other medical conditions. PTAs must be aware of these problems and not only understand how to treat them, but also use their knowledge to prevent them. A PT might not outline each exercise but simply write "therapeutic exercise" in the plan of care. It will then be up to the PTA to think about potential contractures and other physical complications and how to avoid or minimize them.

PTAs use their knowledge of therapeutic exercise to select exercises to minimize muscle atrophy and deconditioning. A physical therapist may order bed mobility and positioning for a geriatric patient who has suffered a severe stroke. The PTA will then need to integrate his or her knowledge of cerebral vascular accidents and bed positioning to determine the best course of action for the patient. When treating geriatric patients, PTAs must constantly think about prevention of complications that may lead to prolonged recoveries.

PTAs must also have sound knowledge and understanding of the psychological and cognitive issues affecting geriatric patients. Although many geriatric patients suffer from conditions such as dementia, Alzheimer's, and other cognitive impairments, PTAs should not assume that all geriatric patients are cognitively impaired. A large number of geriatric patients have little to no cognitive impairment. PTAs need to remember this when treating patients and make sure to use appropriate verbal cues and tone.

With those geriatric patients who do have cognitive impairments, PTAs must understand the patient's cognitive limitations and adjust the treatment accordingly. For instance, a patient with severe cognitive impairment may require simple verbal cues and may not be able to be left alone. PTAs must understand what impact the cognitive impairment will have on the patient's physical therapy. This is not to say that patients with cognitive issues do not receive physical therapy or that they do not improve. On the contrary, patients with cognitive deficits can make amazing gains if they are given appropriate instructions in the proper environment. PTAs must make clinical decisions about how to most effectively communicate and modify the therapy environment to overcome these obstacles.

Besides cognitive problems, patients can become confused and disoriented due to medications or unfamiliar surroundings. Once again, the PTA may decide to alter the patient's treatment as appropriate. In addition to using simple verbal cues, the PTA might decide to treat the patient in the morning, if that is when the patient is most oriented, or to treat the patient in a quieter part of the gym.

PTAs must understand that geriatric patients may experience psychosocial stressors directly related to aging, such as the loss of a spouse or a gradual loss of independence. Such stressors may lead to feelings of depression and inattention to rehabilitation goals. PTAs working with geriatric patients must remain vigilant in detecting psychosocial changes and should report them to the supervising physical therapist. At the same time, PTAs must use their knowledge and understanding of psychological conditions to provide more effective treatment. Oftentimes, this involves using their knowledge to come up with creative ways to motivate the patient to fully participate in therapy.

It can be easy to blame a geriatric patient's lack of participation, motivation, or progress on psychosocial or physiological age-related changes. However, effective PTAs will use their knowledge of geriatric patients in general and the specific patient in particular to devise comprehensive and innovative therapeutic regimens within the scope of the plan of care. Effective PTAs do not give every geriatric patient with a hip fracture the same exercises, but treat each patient as a person with individual needs.

◀ Limits on Clinical Decisions

Treatment plans for geriatric patients tend to emphasize function and are usually less, rather than more, prescriptive. More detailed plans of care are written in cases where there are specific treatment precautions or complicated medical conditions. Treatment plans tend to call for functional activities such as positioning, bed mobility, transfer and ambulation training, as well as therapeutic exercise. Clinical decisions regarding the type of transfer or assistive device or specific exercise regimens are often left to the PTA. Once again, these decisions should be based on sound knowledge and understanding of this distinctive population as well as constant assessment of the patient's condition.

◖ References

Bertoti, D. B. (2004). *Functional Neurorehabilitation Through the Life Span*. Philadelphia, PA: F.A. Davis.

Dreeben, O. (2007). *Introduction to Physical Therapy for Physical Therapist Assistants*. Sudbury, MA: Jones and Bartlett Publishers.

Pagliarulo, M. A. (2007). *Introduction to Physical Therapy* (3rd ed.). St. Louis, MO: Mosby Elsevier.

What Do YOU Think?

▶ **Scenario 1 (Level I)**

Patient is a 75-year-old female who had a left CVA one week ago. The patient is a housewife who lives with her husband in a private home. She babysits her grandson two days a week.

1. You enter the patient's room today and she is crying. What would you do?
2. Describe the psychosocial issues this patient may be experiencing.

▶ **Scenario 2 (Level II)**

Patient is a 70-year-old female with a diagnosis of cancer. She is in the hospital for an acute case of pneumonia and is experiencing severe weakness and pain throughout her body. She is pleasant with the nurses and doctors, but when someone from physical therapy enters the room the patient becomes difficult.

1. Describe the psychosocial issues this patient may be experiencing.
2. Describe how you might best approach this patient.

Level I Activity

▶ **Physical Therapy Evaluation**

Patient is an 80-year-old female s/p right total hip arthroplasty (THA) one week ago secondary to osteoarthritis. THA surgery was done by a posterior approach, cemented. Pt. is WBAT on the right LE. Pt. was admitted to an inpatient rehabilitation center. Pt. is being seen for PT.

PMH: Right shoulder arthroscopy, osteoarthritis, left THA in 2005.

MEDS: Percocet

SH: Pt. lives with her family in a home with many steps without a railing. Prior to admission, pt. was independent in ADLs and amb. with a straight cane secondary to hip pain.

Mental Status: Pt. is alert and oriented ×3. Pt. is able to follow commands without difficulty.

ROM: Bilateral UE and LE are WFL throughout except right shoulder flex 0 to 160 degrees, shoulder abd. 0 to 140 degrees and left hip flex. 0 to 100 degrees, IR/ER 0 to 10 degrees. Right hip flex is 0 to 60 degrees and abd. 0 to 10 degrees secondary to complaints of pain. Right hip IR/ER and ext. not assessed due to pt.'s pain.

Muscle Strength: Bilateral UE and LE are G throughout except right hip not fully assessed secondary to pain.

Sensation: Pt.'s sensation to light touch is intact throughout.

Pain: Pt. with complaints of mild joint stiffness throughout especially in the right shoulder. Pt. complains of pain in the right hip with movement, 8/10 on the pain scale.

Muscle Tone: Pt. displays no abnormal muscle tone.

Balance: Sitting balance—normal. Standing—pt. is able to stand with CG.

Functional Status: Pt. is able to roll to the right with min. assist. Pt. transfers supine ←→ sit with mod. assist, sit ←→ stand with mod. assist. Pt. amb. with right LE WBAT with walker for 20 feet with mod. assist. Pt. has difficulty WB status.

Problems: Pain, decreased active movement, decreased strength, decreased balance, dependency in functional skills.

Short-Term Goals: Pt.'s right hip ROM will increase 10 degrees. Pt. will transfer supine ←→ sit with CG and sit ←→ stand with min. assist. Pt. will amb. with the appropriate assistive device 100 feet with right LE WBAT with min. assist. Pt. will be independent in TH precautions.

Long-Term Goals: Pt. will be independent in transfers. Pt. will ambulate with an appropriate assist device with supervision on level surfaces and on stairs.

Assessment: Pt. is motivated and very cooperative. Pt. appears to be a good rehab. candidate.

Plan: Daily PT for therapeutic exercise, bed mobility, transfers, and ambulation training.

Precautions: THA precautions.

Activity: Patient was evaluated by the physical therapist on her last visit. Perform a treatment and write a progress note. Complete the following questions.
1. Describe the rationale for the exercises you selected.
2. If this patient is being discharged in two weeks, describe some of the discharge needs of this patient.

Level I Activity

▶ **Physical Therapy Evaluation**
Patient Name: _____

HPI: Pt. is an 80-year-old male with Alzheimer's disease and s/p right hip fracture two weeks ago. Pt.'s hospital stay was complicated by a wound infection following surgery. Pt. is continuing his IV antibiotic in this facility. Pt. is WBAT on right LE. Pt. was admitted to an inpatient rehab center two days ago deconditioned. Pt. verbalization is minimal. Pt. is being seen for PT.

PMH: HTN, Alzheimer's disease

MEDS: Lopressor

SH: Pt. lives with his daughter in a ground floor apartment with two steps to enter with a railing. Prior to admission, pt. required constant supervision and minimal assist with ADLs. Prior to admission, pt. ambulated with a walker. Pt.'s daughter is unsure whether she is going to be able to take pt. home upon d/c.

Mental Status: Pt. is alert and is able to follow simple commands.

ROM: Bilateral UE and LE are WFL.

Muscle Strength: Bilateral UE and LE at least F, unable to assess further secondary to mental status.

Sensation: Unable to assess secondary to mental status.

Pain: Pt. does not appear to be in any pain but unable to fully assess secondary to mental status.

Balance: Sitting balance—is able to sit unsupported. Standing balance—pt. is able to maintain static standing with mod. assist.

Functional Status: Pt. requires min-mod. assist for bed mobility. Pt. transfers supine ←→ sit with max. assist, w/c ←→ bed with mod. assist, sit ←→ stand with mod. assist. Pt. amb. right LE WBAT for 5 feet with rolling walker with mod. assist to control balance and walker.

Problems: Decreased balance, dependency in functional skills.

Short-Term Goals: Pt. will perform bed mobility with min. assist—CG. Pt. will transfer supine ←→ sit with min. assist and w/c ←→ bed with min. assist. Pt. will amb. with a rolling walker for 60 feet with right LE WBAT with min. assist.

Long-Term Goals: Pt. will perform all transfers with CG. Pt. will ambulate with an appropriate assist device with CG on level surfaces and on stairs.

Assessment: Pt. appears to be a fair rehabilitation candidate due to the fact that prior to admission pt. only required minimal assist and due to the fact that pt. is able to follow simple commands.

Plan: Daily PT for therapeutic exercise, transfers, and ambulation training.

Activity: Patient was evaluated by the physical therapist at his last visit. Perform a treatment and write a progress note. Complete the following questions.

1. How does this patient's past medical history affect your treatment?
2. Describe some effective communication techniques you could use with this patient.

Level II Activity

▶ **Physical Therapy Evaluation**
Patient Name: _____

HPI: Pt. is an 80-year-old male s/p left CVA one week ago resulting in right hemiparesis. During pt.'s hospital stay pt. suffered a mild MI, but is now cardiac stable. Pt. was admitted to inpatient rehabilitation. Pt. is being seen for PT, OT, and speech therapy.

MH: HTN; OA throughout, especially in the left shoulder.

MEDS: Capoten, Coumadin

SH: Pt. lives alone in an apartment with five steps to enter. Stairs have a railing on the right side. Prior to admission pt. was independent in ADLs.

Mental Status: Pt. is alert and oriented ×3. Pt. is able to follow commands without difficulty.

Vital Signs: Resting HR 68 bpm, BP 130/76 mmHg, Respiration 20 resp./min.

ROM: Left UE and LE are WFL throughout except left shoulder flexion 0 to 110 degrees, abduction 0 to 100 degrees. Pt. displays right UE and LE PROM WFL throughout.

Muscle Strength: Left UE and LE are normal throughout except left shoulder flex and abd are F+. Unable to assess patient's right UE and LE secondary to increased muscle tone.

Sensation: Pt. has decreased sensation to light touch on the right LE.

Pain: Pt. with complaints of mild joint stiffness throughout. Pt. complains of chronic pain in the left shoulder with movements above his head.

Muscle Tone: Pt. displays mild spasticity on the right, UE > LE. Pt. displays a flexor synergy at the right UE and extensor synergy at the right LE. Pt. displays no isolated movement on the right.

Balance: Sitting balance—normal. Standing—pt. is unable to stand independently.

Functional Status: Pt. is able to roll independently. Pt. transfers supine ←→ sit with min. assist, sit ←→ stand with mod. assist. Pt. stood in the parallel bars with mod. assist to support the left side. Pt. with difficulty weight shifting. Pt. able to amb. two steps in the parallel bars with mod. assist to weight shift and min. assist to advance right LE. Pt. displays increased extensor tone at the right LE when ambulating.

Problems: Decreased active movement, decreased strength, abnormal muscle tone, decreased balance, dependency in functional skills.

Short-Term Goals: Pt. will transfer supine ←→ sit with CG and sit ←→ stand with min. assist. Pt. will amb. with the appropriate assistive device 10 feet with mod. assist for balance and weight shifting.

Long-Term Goals: Pt. will be independent in transfers. Pt. will ambulate with an appropriate assist device with supervision on level surfaces and on stairs.

Assessment: Pt. is motivated and very cooperative. Pt. appears to be a good rehab. candidate.

Plan: Daily PT for therapeutic exercise, balance training, bed mobility, transfers, and ambulation training.

Activity: Patient was evaluated by the physical therapist upon his last visit. Perform a treatment and write a progress note. Complete the following questions.
1. How will the patient's recent MI impact patient treatment?
2. Describe the therapeutic exercises that could be performed to decrease the patient's muscle tone.

Clinical Decision Making in Prosthetic and Orthotic Training

11

Prosthetic and orthotic training can be quite complex. Many factors must be attended to simultaneously. The opportunities for PTA clinical decision making are many. However, effective PTAs recognize their limitations. PTAs must strive to be excellent PTAs—not substitute physical therapists. The complexity of prosthetic and orthotic training necessitates effective collaboration between the assistant and therapist.

Physical therapist assistants may be called upon to provide orthotic and prosthetic training. Patients who require orthotic and prosthetic devices vary in age, diagnosis, and functional abilities. Although they do not make the clinical decision to order these devices or select the type of device that best suits a patient, PTAs will make clinical decisions in the training of patients with orthotic and prosthetic devices. These decisions often begin before the patient even receives these devices and continues through the patient's functional or independent use.

◀ Goals of Treatment

Therapeutic goals in orthotic and prosthetic training vary based on the phase of rehabilitation. Preorthotic and preprosthetic training is performed to prepare the patients for their devices. Goals for patients awaiting orthotics may include functional activities—such as gait training—as well as improving range of motion and strength. Preprosthetic training goals may include wound management, shaping of the residual limb, contracture prevention, strengthening, improved range of motion, and functional activities. Once patients have received their orthotic or prosthetic device, goals may advance to functional activities with the devices, including donning and doffing the device, ADL training, and ameliorating gait deviations.

Ultimately, the goal is to ensure safe and independent use of the device. PTAs are only able to make prudent clinical decisions about therapeutic activities if they are aware of the specific goals associated with the orthotic/prosthetic prescription. The types of devices and components differ, and PTAs do not need to be device experts. However, they must exhibit a keen awareness of their patients' impairments and how the prosthetic or orthotic device is designed to improve function.

Goals for patients with amputations will not only depend on the phase of recovery, but also on the patient's age, diagnosis, past medical history, functional abilities, and personal goals. For example, consider two patients: a 21-year-old patient who has undergone a traumatic amputation and a 75-year-old patient who has had an amputation secondary to peripheral vascular disease (PVD). Based on their individual needs, each patient will receive a very different prosthetic device. However, both patients will need a plan of care that involves strengthening and functional training with their new device.

Although less prescriptive treatment plans may appear similar, individual goals may differ. The patient with the traumatic amputation may want to be able to run or ride a bike with his or her prosthesis, whereas the patient with PVD may have less ambitious goals. Although the plan of care for both of these patients may include (pre)prosthetic training, based on each patient's personal goals, age, and other factors the PTA must make important clinical decisions about the types of activities and the intensity of exercise. Goals may also be influenced by the patient's past medical history. Diabetes as well as cardiac and renal disease, for example, will impact the patient's recovery, expected outcomes, and selection of therapeutic activities. PTAs need to consider the whole patient and be able to combine all information when making clinical decisions as to appropriate therapeutic activities.

Orthotic devices vary just as much as the patients who wear them. There are foot orthoses, ankle–foot orthoses, knee–ankle–foot orthoses, as well as trunk and upper extremity orthoses. Patients require orthoses for a variety of reasons, ranging from foot deformities to quadriplegia. Specific goals are adjusted based on the patient's problem and functional abilities. However, all goals focus on the patient becoming as independent as possible. PTAs use their knowledge of different devices and pathologies to fully understand patient goals.

No matter which type of orthotic or prosthetic device the patient receives, goals usually address donning/doffing the device. Another goal may address caring for the device and maintaining skin integrity. The part of the therapeutic plan that coincides with this education may simply be listed as "patient education." PTAs need to make clinical decisions as to what the patient must understand about the device, including proper use, care of the device, and skin care, as well as selecting the best methods by which to teach the patient.

◀ Attendance to Environment

As mentioned earlier, patients requiring orthotic or prosthetic devices are seen in all types of healthcare facilities. Different stages in the recovery process require varying levels of rehabilitation care. PTAs need to be aware of the different stages of the rehabilitation process. For instance, postamputation patients in acute or subacute facilities, require therapeutic emphasis on bed mobility and transfers, ambulating with a walker, and maintenance of range of motion and strength. Effective PTAs recognize the importance of teaching contracture prevention and residual limb shaping using shrinker garments or wrapping techniques (Lusardi and Nielsen, 2007). Clinicians must realize that during the acute/subacute stages patients must adjust to a significantly changed lifestyle. PTAs must make the clinical decision to place a high premium on teaching behavior that ensures patient compliance, progression, and safety.

Patients who have suffered CVAs, TBIs, and other pathologies may display temporary or permanent motor impairment or gait deficits and require orthotic devices. In the very early stages of recovery, it is often too early to order an orthotic device. The physical therapist may decide to use temporary departmental devices. PTAs need to understand the importance of facilitating motion and preventing contractures in order to prepare the patient for the next step in the rehabilitation process.

The next step in rehabilitation may occur in a rehabilitation or nursing home facility. Hopefully, at this point patients are aware of any precautions, know how to avoid contractures, and understand the overall recovery process. PTAs need to remain vigilant in providing appropriate patient education so that the patient will be prepared for the orthotic or prosthetic device. It is at this point that most orthotic and prosthetic devices are ordered.

Delivery of the prosthetic and orthotic devices may occur while the patient is in a rehabilitation center or a nursing home facility or while receiving home care or outpatient physical therapy. When making clinical decisions, PTAs need to consider the patient's current environment. Patient needs and goals will depend on the world around them. For example, a patient in an extended care facility will not need to negotiate the outside environment like someone who is living at home and who must get back and forth to an outpatient physical therapy office. Therefore, goals are appropriately adjusted.

◖ Understanding Patient Needs

As mentioned earlier, patient needs differ based on the stage of the rehabilitation process. Patients requiring prosthetic and orthotic devices may experience a number of psychological issues throughout their recovery. For instance, a patient who has undergone an amputation may struggle with feelings of grief over the loss of the limb. The patient may become depressed and appear unmotivated during treatment. Another patient may have a hard time accepting the reality of the amputation and be too fearful to even look at the residual limb. Still other patients may express anxiety about the recovery process and the use of a prosthetic device. Some patients with amputations develop phantom limb pain. Many patients do not understand that these sensations are common (Lusardi and Nielsen, 2007).

PTAs are not expected to treat patients' psychological problems. However, they are expected to have an understanding of them. When making clinical decisions, PTAs need to take these psychosocial issues into account. For instance, say that a PTA is treating a patient with a recent transtibial amputation who needs to learn how to wrap the residual limb. Normally, this would not be a problem, except that this patient refuses to look at or touch his residual limb. What is the PTA to do? First, the PTA should find out why the patient is refusing to look at the limb and then explain to the patient what it looks like. Next, the PTA could begin teaching wrapping or donning a shrinker using a prop—perhaps a 10–pound sandbag or towel/sheet roll. At the same time, the PTA needs to move the patient toward understanding the importance of looking at and touching the limb so that self-care can progress.

Many of the fears and anxieties patients have are due to their lack of understanding of the recovery process. How long does the limb take to heal? When will they get their prosthesis? Will they ever walk again? These are only some of the questions that may be running through the patients' minds. Although some patients may verbalize these questions, others will hide them under fear and anxiety. PTAs must understand the enormous need for patient education and make the clinical decision to provide the appropriate information and support. PTAs must also attempt to understand the psychological issues patients face and continually try to motivate them by focusing on their abilities rather than their disabilities. Clearly, the overwhelming majority of PTAs have not personally experienced an extremity amputation. However, the decision to maintain an empathetic nature and an understanding of the physical and emotional challenges is critical to the provision of quality care.

Patients with orthotic devices also need education. Patients require orthotics for a number of reasons and need to understand how important these devices are to their overall function. Some patients may be very resistant to wearing orthotics because they are afraid of how they are going to look. This may be especially true of children and adolescents. Older patients may have difficulty accepting a new disability. In either case, PTAs need to understand these patient concerns and provide encouragement and patient education. It is also important to understand the patient's goals as they relate to this new device.

◀ Utilization and Assessment of Objective Measures

When it comes to prosthetic and orthotic devices, the physical therapist will evaluate the patient and determine his or her needs. Ordering of devices is often accomplished through the collaboration of a team consisting of therapy personnel, device specialists, and physicians. Determination of the device type and modification is based on an objective measurement of the patient's status.

It is imperative that PTAs continuously assess their patients throughout all phases of the rehabilitation process. In the early phases of the rehabilitation process, PTAs routinely monitor patients' ROM, strength, edema, pain, and function. Limitations in ROM can affect a patient's ability to use prosthetic or orthotic devices. Changes in strength can affect the type of device the patient needs. Edema may affect the fit of the device. Pain may affect whether the patient wears the device. A change in any one of these factors warrants PT attention (**Figures 11.1** and **11.2**). Goniometry, manual muscle testing, circumferential measurement, and other objective assessment techniques must be regularly employed.

Integument	• Excessive or protracted redness • Skin breakdown • Edema monitoring
Proper fit	• Suspension • Excessive rotation • Excessive pistoning • Pain complaint • Edema monitoring
Gait deviations	• Medial/Lateral whip • Circumduction • Hip hike

Figure 11.1 Common Prosthetic Monitoring Considerations

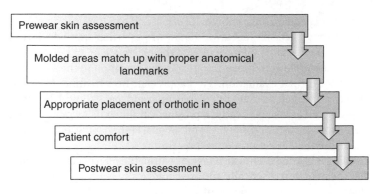

Figure 11.2 Common Orthotic Monitoring Considerations

When providing orthotic and prosthetic training, PTAs must closely monitor the patient's skin condition. Regardless of the stage of recovery, skin breakdown significantly retards rehabilitation. Skin integrity assessment begins at the initial evaluation and continues throughout the rehabilitation process. The use of careful observation, tape measures, transparent grids, and digital analyzers is critical to sound monitoring. Once patients receive their prosthetic or orthotic device, objective assessment and monitoring continue. Initially, the physical therapist will assess fit and function of the device. However, effective PTAs are vigilant in monitoring potential changes in fit. Such changes are immediately reported to the supervising therapist.

◖ Possession of Sound Clinical Knowledge and Expertise

Clearly, a sound knowledge of the pathologies that precipitate the need for orthotics and prosthetics is crucial to effective management. Effective PTAs make clinical decisions based on this knowledge. They maintain a basic understanding of the potential and multiple seque-lae that are associated with prosthetic and orthotic use. For instance, in the case of lower extremity devices, effective PTAs are mindful of closed kinetic chain considerations. They understand that changes in one portion of the kinetic chain—precipitated by the device—cause changes up and down the chain.

PTAs depend on their knowledge of gait and make appropriate clinical decisions. PTAs may not always know why a particular gait deviation exists, but effective PTAs recognize the existence of gait deviations and make the clinical decision to report the deviation to the supervising PT for further evaluation. They appreciate how treatment emphasis differs based on the stage of rehabilitation and make clinical decisions accordingly. For instance, early in prosthetic training PTAs must exhibit more expertise with and emphasis on residual limb shaping, edema control techniques, and contracture prevention.

PTAs must make clinical decisions within the plan of care to ensure that the patient is physically and psychologically ready for the device. Once again, in the presence of a less prescriptive plan PTAs must stand ready to make basic clinical decisions about important aspects of physical management, including type of exercise, muscular group emphasis, and teaching strategies. These basic clinical decisions require sound clinical knowledge and expertise.

PTAs must not only know the importance of proper fitting prosthetic and orthotic devices, but also know the signs that indicate that the device is not fitting properly. Any concerns regarding the fit of the prosthetic or orthotic device must be reported to the supervising physical therapist.

◀ Limits on Clinical Decisions

Prosthetic and orthotic training can be quite complex. Many factors must be attended to simultaneously. The opportunities for PTA clinical decision making are many. However, effective PTAs recognize their limitations. PTAs must strive to be excellent PTAs—not substitute physical therapists. The complexity of prosthetic and orthotic training necessitates effective collaboration between the assistant and therapist.

◀ References

Edelstein, J. E., & Bruckner, J. (2002). *Orthotics: A Comprehensive Clinical Approach.* Thorofar, NJ: Slack.

Lusardi, M. M., & Nielsen, C. C. (2007). *Orthotics and Prosthetics in Rehabilitation* (2nd ed.). St. Louis, MO: Saunders Elsevier.

What Do YOU Think?

▶ **Scenario 1 (Level II)**

The patient is a 75-year-old woman recovering from a left transtibial amputation performed three days ago. She is currently awaiting inpatient rehabilitation in an acute care hospital.

   1. What are the patient's education needs at this time?

   2. Describe the patient education you would perform regarding proper positioning.

▶ **Scenario 2 (Level II)**

The patient is a 70-year-old woman recovering from a left transtibial amputation. She received her prosthesis approximately two weeks ago. When the patient ambulates, you notice that during swing the patient displays increased hip flexion. What might be the possible causes of this increased hip flexion? What can be done about it?

▶ **Scenario 3 (Level II)**

Your patient has a left transfemoral prosthetic device. When the patient ambulates you notice that he circumducts his left lower extremity. During what phase of gait would you expect to see the circumduction? What might be one possible cause?

Level I Activity

▶ **Physical Therapy Evaluation**

The patient is a 45-year-old male recovering from left transtibial amputation three days ago. At present, the patient is in an acute care facility.

PMH: DM, HTN, OA

SH: Pt. lives alone in an apartment with 15 steps to enter.

Mental Status: Pt. is A&O × 3.

ROM: Bil. UE and LE WFL throughout except left hip flexion −25 to 120 degrees and left knee flexion −20 to 130 degrees.

Strength: Bil. UE G; R LE G; L LE hip flexion F−, ext P, abd. P+, add. P, IR/ER F, knee flex/ext. F.

Sensation: Intact in response to light touch throughout.

Pain: Complaints of phantom leg pain.

Transfers: Pt. transfers supine → sit independently, sit → stand with min. assist.

Ambulation: Pt. hops with walker for 20 feet with minimal assist for balance.

Balance: Sitting—static/dynamic normal. Standing—static F and dynamic F−.

Problems: Dec. ROM, dec. strength, dependency in transfers and ambulation.

Goals: STG: Pt. will transfer sit → stand with supervision; pt. will ambulate with walker for 50 feet with standby assist.

LTG: Pt.'s range of motion will increase 10 degrees to prepare for prosthesis. Pt.'s strength will increase a half grade in preparation for prosthesis.

Assessment: Pt. appears to be a good inpatient rehabilitation candidate. He is cooperative and eager for his prosthesis.

Plan: Daily PT for ROM, strength, transfers, balance training, ambulation, and residual limb care, including wrapping and desensitization and proper positioning.

Activity: Perform a treatment on the patient and write a progress note regarding the patient's treatment. Answer the following questions.

1. List two exercises you would perform with this patient and describe the rationale for each.

2. Describe one activity that could be done to improve this patient's balance.
3. Discuss the psychosocial issues this patient may be experiencing at this time and what you can do as a PTA.

Level II Activity

▶ **Physical Therapy Evaluation**

The patient described in the previous activity is now eight weeks post op and is in an outpatient facility. The patient has just received his new prosthesis. The following is the physical therapy evaluation in the outpatient facility.

PMH: DM, HTN, OA

SH: Pt. lives alone in an apartment with 15 steps to enter.

Mental Status: Pt. is A&O ×3.

ROM: Bil. UE and LE WFL throughout.

Strength: Bil. UE G; R LE G; L LE G.

Sensation: Intact in response to light touch throughout.

Pain: Complaints of occasional phantom leg pain.

Prosthesis: Pt. has a transtibial prosthesis. Pt. requires assist to don/doff prosthesis.

Transfers: Pt. transfers supine → sit → stand independently.

Ambulation: Pt. hops with walker for 20 feet independently. Ambulated the length of the parallel bars with prosthesis with mod. assist for balance and coordination.

Balance: Sitting—static/dynamic normal. Standing with prosthesis—static/dynamic F.

Problems: Dec. ROM, dec. strength, dependency in transfers and ambulation.

Goals: STG: Pt. will don/doff prosthesis independently. Pt. will ambulate with prosthesis 3× the length of the parallel bars with CG—min. assist for balance.

LTG: Pt. will ambulate with his prosthesis with an appropriate assistive device on level and uneven surfaces independently. Pt. will be independent in the care of his residual and prosthesis.

Assessment: Pt. appears to be a good outpatient rehabilitation candidate. He is cooperative and eager to learn how to ambulate with his prosthesis.

Plan: Daily PT for ROM, strength, transfers, balance training, ambulation, and prosthetic training, including donning and doffing.

Activity: Perform a treatment on the patient and write a progress note regarding the patient's treatment. Answer the following questions.

1. What are the patient's education needs with regards to using a prosthetic device?
2. What type of assistive device would you start with once the patient leaves the parallel bars? Explain.
3. What type of balance activities could you do with this patient at this time?

Level II Activity

▶ Physical Therapy Evaluation

We continue with the same patient as in the previous two activities. Our patient has returned to the hospital one year later and has undergone a right transfemoral amputation. The patient is currently receiving physical therapy in an inpatient rehabilitation facility.

PMH: DM, HTN, OA, left transtibial amputation.

SH: Pt. lives alone in an apartment with 15 steps to enter. Pt. states he has been unable to wear his prosthesis for the past year secondary to a decubiti he developed on the distal end of his left LE.

Mental Status: Pt. is A&O ×3.

ROM: Bil. UE and LE WFL throughout except right hip flexion 0 to 90 degrees and add. 0 to 5 degrees.

Strength: Bil. UE G; L LE G; R LE hip flex. F, ext. P, abd. P–, add. P–, IR/ER P.

Sensation: Intact in response to light touch throughout.

Pain: Complaints of bilateral phantom leg pain.

Transfers: Pt. is independent in bed mobility and transfers supine → sit with contact guard and transfers OOB → chair with max. assist ×2.

Balance: Sitting—static G dynamic F.

Problems: Dec. ROM, dec. strength, dependency in transfers.

Goals: STG: Pt. will be independent in wrapping of right residual limb. Pt. will transfer supine → sit independently. Pt. will transfer OOB → chair with a sliding board transfer with mod. assist.

LTG: Pt.'s right LE strength will increase a half grade. Pt.'s ROM will increase 5 degrees. Pt. will transfer OOB → wheelchair independently with sliding board. Pt. will be independent in wheelchair mobility on level surfaces.

Plan: Daily physical therapy for ROM, strengthening, transfer training, and wheelchair mobility.

Activity: Perform a treatment on the patient and write a progress note regarding the patient's treatment. Answer the following questions.

1. Why was a sliding board transfer selected for this patient?
2. What wheelchair mobility activities will you teach this patient?
3. What problems may this patient face if he is discharged to his home?

Clinical Decision Making in Managing Patients with Complex Acute Medical Conditions

12

Patients receiving critical care are surrounded by and attached to a wide array of medical and monitoring devices. The number of tubes, lines, and wires that appear to emerge from all parts of the patient's body, as well as the audible whirs and alarms of medical devices, present a daunting sight for PTAs. PTAs must develop a comfort level in providing physical therapy interventions in this environment. In order to competently provide physical therapy care, PTAs must become familiar with the medical devices common to this environment.

Oftentimes, PTAs employed in inpatient acute care facilities are called upon to provide physical therapy care to patients presenting with complex diagnoses, postsurgical conditions, significant debilitation, and multiple sequelae. These services—at least initially—are often provided at the bedside. Patients receiving these services may be in critical care units or medical–surgical units. Ideally, PTAs providing care to this patient population are teamed with physical therapists. Together, the PT and PTA manage a caseload of patients who are critically ill or in early postoperative phases of recovery.

When providing services to these patients, PTAs are often faced with a wide array of infusion lines, monitors, alarms, and patient complaints of pain and discomfort. To the novice PTA, in particular, this therapeutic scene may be intimidating—even frightening. The perceived anxiety is overcome by gaining a sound understanding of patients' medical needs and monitoring requirements. Open communication with and guidance from the supervising PT and nursing personnel are crucial. Physical therapy intervention during these early stages of recovery may facilitate the success of future rehabilitation. PTAs must quickly overcome their anxieties and stand ready to provide safe and high-quality physical therapy interventions.

In providing physical therapy care to critically ill patients, PTAs must make a variety of clinical decisions related to the type and intensity of the provided interventions. These clinical decisions are significantly influenced by a patient's medical status, as measured by vital signs, serum levels, pharmacologic interactions, physical condition, and so on. PTAs must be sensitive to these variables. They must be able to readily discern abnormal values and recognize adverse physical signs that may hamper attainment of therapeutic goals. Early in the recovery process, a patient's physical condition may change from day to day. PTAs must vigilantly match chosen interventions with the patient's present condition. Given these patients' often fragile medical status, PTAs must ensure that chosen physical therapy interventions are directly linked with the treatment goals.

◀ Treatment Goals

Physical therapy intervention for critically ill patients typically commences at the bedside. The presence of multiple infusion lines and monitors, as well as the patient's debilitated physical condition and need for close medical supervision, precludes transportation from the medical unit. Physical therapy goals during this phase of rehabilitation necessarily revolve around basic function and the prevention of complications associated with protracted bed rest and debilitation. These goals include: (1) maintenance and improvement of pulmonary status, (2) facilitation of bed mobility, (3) maintenance and improvement of joint range of motion, (4) maintenance and improvement of muscle strength and endurance, and (5) facilitation of sit-to-stand transfers and early gait (**Figure 12.1**).

PTAs must make the clinical decision to carefully prioritize interventions. For instance, when providing service to a heavily sedated and somewhat lethargic patient the PTA may make the clinical decision to concentrate on preventive interventions, such as PROM and

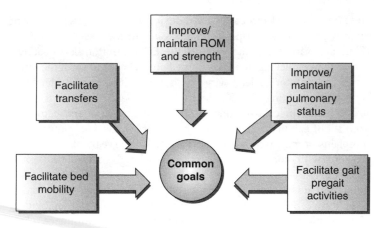

Figure 12.1 Common Goals for Patients with Complex Acute Medical Conditions

stretching activities, gradually progressing to more active interventions as the patient's medical condition improves. Similarly, based on a patient's complaint of discomfort or the completion of an invasive procedure, the PTA—rather than not providing physical therapy care—may decide to provide less aggressive interventions.

◀ Attendance to the Environment

Patients receiving critical care are surrounded by and attached to a wide array of medical and monitoring devices. The number of tubes, lines, and wires that appear to emerge from all parts of the patient's body, as well as the audible whirs and alarms of medical devices, present a daunting sight for PTAs. PTAs must develop a comfort level in providing physical therapy interventions in this environment. In order to competently provide physical therapy care, PTAs must become familiar with the medical devices common to this environment.

The placement of central and other intravenous (IV) lines, the presence of electrocardiogram (ECG) monitoring electrodes, or the placement of a nasogastric (NG) tube certainly influence clinical decisions as to how interventions are provided or how the PTA reacts to warning alarms. For instance, say that a patient in a critical care unit is being monitored by an electrocardiogram device. A PTA enters the patient room with the intent of performing PROM to the lower extremities. While performing the intervention, the ECG monitor alarm sounds. Rather than panicking, the PTA immediately checks to see if the lower extremity monitoring lead wire has become dislodged. By having a basic understanding of ECG electrode placement, the PTA is better able to make clinical decisions. Similarly, say that a patient recovering from a TBI exhibits a change in behavior or relative consciousness or complains of increased headache. The PTA observes that intracranial pressure (ICP) monitoring is in place and makes the clinical decision to check the ICP—normal ICP is 4 to 15 mmHg—or to alert nursing personnel and the supervising PT of the change in the patient's presentation (O'Sullivan & Schmitz, 2007). Here again, it is the PTA's understanding of the monitoring devices within the environment that influences clinical decisions. **Table 12.1** describes some common devices used in managing patients with acute medical conditions.

Table 12.1 Common Medical Equipment and Devices Used in Managing Patients with Acute Medical Conditions

Device	Description	Comments
Central line	Intravenous catheter passed through a peripheral vessel and ending in the vena cava. Allows for better infusion of concentrated solutions and monitoring of vessel pressures.	Increased risk of infection with certain types of central lines. Potential infiltration if tubing disconnected improperly.
Electrocardiogram (ECG/EKG)	Mechanical device that monitors electrical activity of the heart via external electrodes placed on the torso and extremities.	The device alarms when electrodes become dislodged or anomalies are detected.
Intracranial pressure (ICP) monitor	Mechanical device that measures intracranial pressure via a surgically implanted pressure sensor.	The device monitors and alarms when intracranial pressure falls outside of normal range.
Intravenous infusion pump	Medical device that controls the infusions of intravenous medication.	The device may alarm when infusion is impaired due to possible infiltration, occlusion, or other reason.
Mechanical ventilator with intubation	Mechanical device that ventilates a patient's lungs via tubing inserted through the mouth and placed in the airway.	The patient is unable to speak or eat when intubated. The patient is at increased risk for pneumonia.
Nasogastric (NG) tube	Feeding tube inserted through the nose and ending in the stomach.	Patient may complain of throat irritation. Possibility of gastric reflux.

◀ Utilization and Assessment of Objective Measures

When making clinical decisions about physical therapy care provided to patients with complex acute medical conditions, PTAs must be very aware and knowledgeable of different objective physiological indices. Even small changes in vital signs, serum electrolyte levels, or complete blood count (CBC) values may significantly affect patient participation in physical therapy activities. For example, say that a PTA is providing physical therapy at the bedside of a 63-year-old woman following a cholecystectomy with postsurgical sepsis. In this case, physical therapy interventions are limited to straight leg raises and weighted-wand exercises for the upper extremities. The PTA notes that over the last two to three visits the patient has been exhibiting increased fatigue and decreased tolerance to treatment. A review of the medical record indicates that over the last three days the patient's red blood cells (RBC) have decreased from 4.2 to 3.8 million/mm³. The decreased value—although just slightly abnormal—may indeed affect the patient's ability to tolerate physical therapy treatment. The PTA may make the clinical decision to alert the supervising PT of the decrease in the RBC count. The wise clinical decision here is not to simply document the patient's decreased tolerance, but to also seek a potential cause based on available objective indicators. **Table 12.2** provides normal complete blood count values and rehabilitation consequences of abnormal values (Skinner & Hurley, 2007). The PTA may also make clinical decisions about a patient's inability to meet goals or tolerate treatment by correlating signs and symptoms with serum electrolyte levels (**Table 12.3**).

When providing physical therapy services to acutely ill patients, PTAs must constantly be aware of the patient's cardiopulmonary status. When signs of respiratory distress arise, PTAs must make the clinical decision to cease treatment and consult the supervising PT and nursing personnel. Cyanosis—a bluish tinge of the skin most easily seen around the mouth and lips and at the nail beds—is a powerful indicator of decreased oxygenation. Its presence is linked to the amount of oxygen bound to circulating hemoglobin and is associated with pulmonary or cardiac compromise (Goodman Cavallaro, Fuller, & Boissonnault, 2003).

Table 12.2 Complete Blood Count (CBC) Values

Assessment Component	Values	Implications/Red Flags
Red blood cells (RBC; erythrocytes)		
Infants	5.5–6.0 million/mm³	Individuals with lower than normal values have anemia.
Children	4.6–4.8 million/mm³	Symptoms of anemia include fatigue, weakness, shortness of breath, dizziness, and tachycardia.
Men	4.5–5.3 million/mm³	Individuals with higher than normal values have polycythemia.
Women	4.1–5.1 million/mm³	Symptoms of polycythemia include shortness of breath, headache, dizziness, and itchiness.
Erythrocyte sedimentation rate (ESR/Sed. Rate)		
Children	1–13 mm/hr	ESR is the rate at which erythrocytes settle out of blood plasma in one hour. A high rate is indicative of infection or inflammation.
Men	0–17 mm/hr	
Women	1–25 mm/hr	
Hematocrit (HCT)		
Infants	30%–60%	Hematocrit is the percent of whole blood composed of erythrocytes. Exercise may be restricted at values ≤25%.
Children	30%–49%	
Men	37%–49%	
Women	36%–46%	
Hemoglobin (HGB)		
Infants	17–19 g/dL	HGB measures the oxygen-carrying capacity of RBCs. Low values (between 8–10 g/dL) are associated with poor exercise tolerance, increased fatigue, and tachycardia.
Children	14–17 g/dL	
Men	13–18 g/dL	
Women	12–16 g/dL	
Platelets		
Infants	200,000–475,000 cells/mm³	Platelets play a key role in initiation of the clotting process within damaged blood vessels.
Children	150,000–400,000 cells/mm³	Exercise may be cautiously performed with values of 21,000–50,000 cells/mm³.
Adults	150,000–400,000 cells/mm³	Exercise may be contraindicated at values ≤20,000 cells/mm³.

(Continued)

Table 12.2 Complete Blood Count (CBC) Values (*Continued*)

White blood cells (WBCs)		
Children	4,500–14,500 cells/mm³	WBCs play a crucial role in the body's immune system.
Adults	4,500–11,000 cells/mm³	Exercise may be contraindicated at values ≤5,000 cells/mm³.
Differential WBC		
Neutrophils	1,800–7,000 cells/mm³	The various WBCs play different roles in the immune response. They exist in stereotypical proportions.
Lymphocytes	1,500–4,000 cells/mm³	
Monocytes	0–800 cells/mm³	
Eosinophils	0–450 cells/mm³	
Basophils	0–200 cells/mm³	

Table 12.3 Serum Electrolyte Values

Electrolyte	Values	Description/Red Flags
Potassium		
Children	3.5–5.5 mEq/L	Symptoms of low potassium (hypokalemia) include dizziness, muscle weakness, fatigue, and leg cramps.
Adults	3.5–5.3 mEq/L	Symptoms of high potassium (hyperkalemia) include muscle weakness, flaccid paralysis, and paresthesias.
Sodium		
	135–145 mEq/L	Symptoms of low sodium (hyponatremia) include muscle twitching and weakness. Symptoms of high sodium (hypernatremia) include fever and convulsions.
Chloride		
Children	98–105 mEq/L	Chloride shifts are most often associated with shifts in sodium.
Adults	95–105 mEq/L	
Calcium		
Children	9–11.5 mg/dL	Symptoms of low calcium (hypocalcemia) include paresthesias and muscle spasms.
Adults	9–11 mg/dL	Symptoms of high calcium (hypercalcemia) include lethargy, muscle weakness, flaccidity, and bone pain.
Magnesium		
Children	1.6–2.6 mEq/L	Symptoms of low magnesium (hypomagnesemia) include muscle cramping, tetany, and confusion.
Adults	1.5–2.5 mEq/L	Symptoms of high magnesium (hypermagnesemia) include decreased reflexes, muscle weakness, and lethargy.

When working with patients at risk for pulmonary compromise, PTAs make the clinical decision to watch for signs of cyanosis. In people with darker skin, cyanosis may not be as readily visible around the mouth and lips. PTAs scanning for cyanosis in this patient population should concentrate on observation of the nail beds. Other signs of respiratory distress include perfuse perspiration (diaphoresis), increased respiratory rate, irregular respiration patterns, inspiratory flaring of the nostrils, and audible respiration (**Figure 12.2**). Signs of respiratory distress

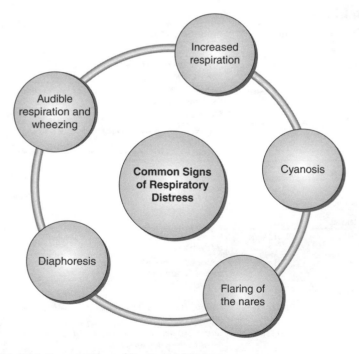

Figure 12.2 Common Signs of Respiratory Distress

may emerge gradually during a therapy session. PTAs must monitor the patient for signs of distress throughout the entire session. When initial signs of distress are observed, a decision to alter or cease therapeutic activities must be made.

In addition to signs of pulmonary distress, PTAs must know the significance of objective vital sign values. Normal values differ with age (Skinner & Hurley, 2007). **Table 12.4** provides normal vital sign values. Pulse and respiratory rate, blood pressure, and oxygen saturation are critical physiological indicators and may clearly be altered by physical therapy intervention. Physical exertion typically increases pulse,

Table 12.4 Normal Vital Sign Values

Vital Sign	Normal Range
Heart rate (pulse)	
Newborn	70–90 beats/min
1 year old	80–160 beats/min
2–6 years old	70–125 beats/min
8–12 years old	70–110 beats/min
13–16 years old	60–100 beats/min
Adults	55–100 beats/min
Blood pressure	
Birth to 1 month	Systolic: 60–90 mmHg Diastolic: 30–60 mmHg
2 months to 3 years	Systolic: 75–130 mmHg Diastolic: 45–90 mmHg
3 years through adult	Systolic: 90–140 mmHg Diastolic: 50–80 mmHg
Respiratory rate	
Birth to 1 month	35–55 breaths/min
3 months to 6 years old	20–30 breaths/min
6–10 years old	15–25 breaths/min
10–16 years old	12–30 breaths/min
Adults	12–20 breaths/min
Oxygen saturation (measured with pulse oximeter)	98% at rest or during exercise. Exercise may be contraindicated at values ≤90%.

respiratory rate, and systolic blood pressure, while oxygen saturation and diastolic pressure remain relatively constant (Goodman Cavallaro, Fuller, & Boissonnault, 2003). By understanding how physical therapy interventions affect vital signs, PTAs are better positioned to make appropriate clinical decisions. For instance, PTAs must monitor blood pressure when initially progressing patients to upright positions of sitting and standing. The presence of orthostatic hypotension—a sudden and prolonged drop in blood pressure with changes in position—precipitates the clinical decision to more slowly progress the patient to the upright position (O'Sullivan & Schmitz, 2007).

◖ Limits on Clinical Decisions

Clinical decisions related to the type or sequence of physical therapy interventions may be significantly influenced by formal protocols. This may be especially true when managing patients recovering from cardiac surgery. Postsurgical protocols typically prescribe a day-by-day sequence of therapeutic activities. However, the use of formal protocols in no way precludes PTAs from making prudent clinical decisions that maintain patient safety. For instance, one postoperative protocol calls for "dangling at the edge of the bed" at post op day 3. However, orthostatic hypotension may force delayed attainment of this goal. Protocols may be strict guidelines, but they do not trump clinical decisions that preserve patient safety.

◖ References

Goodman Cavallaro, C., Fuller, K. S., & Boissonnault, W. G. (2003). *Pathology: Implications for the Physical Therapist* (2nd ed.). Philadelphia, PA: Saunders.

O'Sullivan, S. B., & Schmitz, T. J. (2007). *Physical Rehabilitation* (5th ed.). Philadelphia, PA: F.A. Davis.

Skinner, S. B., & Hurley, C. (2007). *Pocket Notes for the Physical Therapist Assistant.* Sudbury, MA: Jones and Bartlett Publishers.

What Do YOU Think?

▶ **Scenario 1 (Level I)**

The patient is a 79-year-old female who presents in the surgical ICU following a partial bowel resection secondary to colorectal cancer. She was referred to physical therapy for ROM, bed mobility, transfer, and pregait activities. Upon entering the room, the PTA notes that the patient's respiratory rate is 14 breaths/min, pulse is 92 beats/min, oxygen saturation is 88%, blood pressure is 138/89 mmHg, and ECG shows normal sinus rhythm. Would straight leg raises and weighted-wand activities to improve strength necessary for transfer and bed mobility activities be appropriate for this patient? Explain.

▶ **Scenario 2 (Level II)**

The patient is a 12-year-old male who has been admitted to the PICU for bacterial meningitis. The patient emerged from a three-day coma two days ago. The patient was referred to PT for bedside therapy for early rehabilitation. The medical record indicates the following values: ESR, 14 mm/hr; HGB, 12 g/dL; WBC, 16,000 cells/mm³; and ICP 14 mmHg. What do these values suggest? What actions should the PTA take?

▶ **Scenario 3 (Level II)**

Your patient is in an acute care hospital following a coronary artery bypass graft one week ago. The patient is independent in functional activities and is being discharged in two days. The PT has ordered a walking program for this patient. What patient education needs to be done with this patient regarding vital signs and a walking program?

▶ **Scenario 4 (Level II)**

Your patient is in an acute care hospital suffering from pneumonia. The physical therapy treatment plan calls for pulmonary toileting and breathing exercises. How would you approach this treatment?

Level I Activity

▶ **Physical Therapy Evaluation**

Patient is a 63-year-old female recovering from a Whipple procedure five days ago. Extubated two days ago. Patient was diagnosed with pancreatic cancer approximately six weeks ago. Patient remains in surgical ICU. Patient referred to PT for bed mobility, transfer, and gait activities.

PMH: HTN

SH: Pt. lives on lower level of two-family home with husband, daughter, and grandchildren.

Mental Status: Pt. is A&O × 3 with frequent episodes of lethargy.

ROM: Patient presents with WFL ROM both UEs. ROM at ankles is WNL. Hip and knee ROM not fully assessed due to complaint of abdominal pain.

Strength: UE strength is 3.5/5 throughout bilaterally. LE not assessed due to c/o abdominal pain.

Other: Pain managed with PCA. Pt. is maintained in semi-Fowler position.

Functional: Pt. requires moderate assist for all bed mobility mainly due to pain. Transfers supine to sit with mod. to max. assist, with pain and c/o dizziness as limiting factors. Sit-to-stand transfer not attempted due to pain and fatigue.

Problems: (1) Abdominal pain, (2) extremity weakness, (3) assisted bed mobility, (4) unable to move sit to stand.

Plan: Daily PT. Interventions to include bed mobility, ROM, strengthening, transfer, and gait activities.

Goals: STG (within two visits): Min. assist bed mobility in all directions, min. assist transfer supine ←→ sit, mod. assist transfers sit ←→ stand.

LTG (within six visits): Independent bed mobility, supervised transfer supine ←→ sit, min. assist sit ←→ stand transfer, contact guard ambulation × 50 feet with walker.

Activity: The patient was evaluated yesterday. Perform a treatment and write a progress note. Answer the following questions.
1. What factors may limit attainment of the patient's therapeutic goals? In response to the identified factors, how would you alter your treatment?
2. Identify a potential cause of the patient's complaint of dizziness.

Level II Activity

▶ **Physical Therapy Evaluation**

Patient is a 31-year-old male who was in a motor vehicle accident four weeks ago resulting in a TBI. Upon admission to the acute care facility, the patient was comatose for three weeks. Patient is now more responsive and alert. Patient has an IV and is on a heart monitor.

PMH: None

SH: Pt. lives alone in a second-floor apartment.

Mental Status: Pt. is able to follow simple commands but is lethargic.

ROM: Bilateral UEs are WNL and LEs are WFL except right DF −10 degrees from neutral.

Strength: Bilateral UEs appear at least Fair strength—difficult to fully assess due to mental status and right LE is good and right LE at hip and knee poor and ankle zero strength.

Sensation: Appears intact to light touch.

Vital Signs: Resting vital signs are within normal limits.

Functional Status: Patient requires moderate assistance for bed mobility.

Problems: Decreased ROM and strength, dependency in bed mobility, and state of alertness.

Goals: STG: Increase right dorsiflexion 5 degrees. Patient will be able to roll side to side with minimal assistance. Patient will dangle on side of bed.

LTG: Patient right dorsiflexion range of motion will be WNL in order to ambulate efficiently. Patient will be independent in bed mobility. Patient will perform transfers with supervision. Patient will ambulate independently with the appropriate assistive device.

Plan: Daily PT for stretching, strengthening, bed mobility, and transfer training.

Activity: This patient was evaluated yesterday. Perform a treatment on this patient, write a SOAP note, and then complete the following questions.

1. What was done to address this patient's lack of range of motion in his ankle? What may be done to prevent further contracture at the ankle?
2. Upon sitting on the side of the bed, the patient fainted. What would you do? How might this be prevented in the future?

Effective PTAs devise ways to effectively compile treatment regimens that comply with the prescribed treatment plan and meet their patients' long-term and immediate needs.

PTAs must be effective case managers. They must synthesize efficacious treatment sessions consistent with the plan of care and patients' needs. Effective PTAs are efficient and thorough readers. They are able to glean important facts from an initial evaluation and immediately begin the process of integrating the provided objective and subjective data into a cohesive treatment regimen. Although the physical therapist's plan of care may delineate specific interventions, it may not spell out exactly how the plan should be implemented. Variables such as sequence of therapeutic activities, emphasis of techniques, and selection of therapeutic activities represent clinical decisions that must be made by the treating clinician. For instance, a therapeutic plan may include "AROM activities" for the shoulder. If not specified, the PTA must decide on the appropriate AROM activities—wand activities, wall climbing, ball throwing, and so on.

It is unrealistic and likely ineffective to assume that patients with similar diagnoses can be treated identically. Subtle—and not so subtle—differences in symptoms, age, mental status, personal goals, and so on mandate the synthesis of customized treatment sessions for each patient.

◀ ORBIT

PTAs devise ways to effectively compile treatment regimens that comply with the prescribed plan of care and meet their patients' long-term and immediate needs. The use of the acronym ORBIT may help PTAs perform this task (**Figure 13.1**). ORBIT represents a three-part decision-making process. The first part of this process is represented by the words *organize*, *relate*, and *bracket*. The second part is represented by the word *integrate*. The third part is represented by the word *treat*.

Organize, Relate, and Bracket

Effective PTAs are acutely aware of their patients' clinical problems. Following review of the initial evaluation, they begin to organize themselves to provide treatment by first—either physically or mentally—devising a patient problem/clinical manifestation list. This list is gleaned from the subjective and objective information contained in the initial evaluation. Compiling this list provides an opportunity for the PTA to better focus on the patient's specific rehabilitation issues and quickly begin the next phase of the clinical decision/management process.

Once the patient's problems have been organized into a list, the PTA begins to relate these problems to each other and to their functional consequences. For instance, a problem list for a patient with CVA may include the following: maximum assist transfers, left lower extremity extensor spasticity, moderately impaired sitting balance, and unsafe ambulation. PTAs may relate the maximum assist transfers and unsafe gait and bracket them together with the left lower extremity spasticity. In other

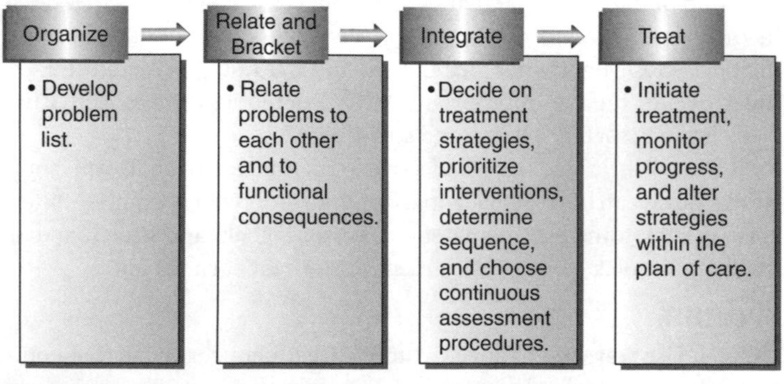

Organize	Relate and Bracket	Integrate	Treat
• Develop problem list.	• Relate problems to each other and to functional consequences.	• Decide on treatment strategies, prioritize interventions, determine sequence, and choose continuous assessment procedures.	• Initiate treatment, monitor progress, and alter strategies within the plan of care.

Figure 13.1 ORBIT Case Management

words, the PTA is in effect stating that the spasticity must be principally addressed in order to improve the bracketed signs and symptoms. A list of problems may be prioritized, related, and bracketed in multiple ways, and rarely is one problem related exclusively to another. However, the process of relating and bracketing clinical manifestations helps set the stage for the synthesis of a therapeutic regimen that is effective and compact.

Integrate

The next step in the ORBIT model is to integrate the processed data into a therapeutic regimen. For instance, given how the clinical manifestations in the previously mentioned patient were organized, related, and bracketed, the PTA may decide to start the treatment session with mat, ROM, and NDT activities to help normalize tone, followed by sitting balance, transfer, and gait activities. During this phase, PTAs may also decide what continuous assessment means they will use to monitor progress. This may be predetermined in the initial evaluation; however, it does not preclude PTAs from using additional assessment measures, if appropriate. Effective PTAs enter into each therapeutic encounter with a well thought out plan of action in mind.

Treat

Having completed the first two steps, PTAs are now ready to treat the patient. By following the steps of the ORBIT model, treatment will occur in a more orderly, efficient, and logical manner. Note that the steps of the ORBIT model do not necessarily require significant time to complete. With experience, PTAs may perform the process as a routine mental exercise before every therapeutic encounter. The goal is for PTAs to avoid falling into the bad habit of providing stereotypical treatments that may not account for the wide array of clinical variability. The proceeding paragraphs provide an application of the ORBIT process.

◀ Application of the ORBIT Model

Here we present excerpts from a physical therapist evaluation of a patient diagnosed with Parkinson's disease. Parkinson's disease is a chronic progressive neurological disease. The etiology of the disease is rooted in abnormalities of the basal ganglia of the brain characterized by a degeneration of neurons that produce dopamine, a neurotransmitter. Major clinical manifestations include bradykinesia, rigidity, and tremor. The excerpted initial evaluation contains stereotypical findings that may be present in an initial evaluation. A PTA can use the ORBIT clinical decision model to fashion a physical therapy session.

Pt. is an alert and oriented 62 y.o. old male s/p Parkinson's disease initially diagnosed two years ago. Pt. has been referred to PT due to an apparent exacerbation of symptoms over the past four months. The patient relates increased "tripping" during gait, inability to walk usual distances due to fatigue, problems performing ADLs due to "freezing in the middle of the activity," increased difficulty getting out of bed and transferring from sit to stand. The patient states that he is trying to remain active. He "walks" every day, either outside or in the local shopping mall. The patient states that he has recently been prescribed Sinemet but is concerned that his symptoms have not rapidly changed.

Mild masked faces is noted. Mild-to-moderate resting tremor of upper extremities is noted. Pt. moves from sit to stand independently. However, maintenance of balance during transfers is mildly impaired and transfers are awkward and slowed. Pt. is noted to ambulate independently without an assistive device. A mild-to-moderate foot drag is noted on the right. Arm swing appears moderately decreased bilaterally. Trunk rotation during gait is moderately impaired. Patient required assistance moving from sit to supine due to coordination impairment, mild freezing, and moderate trunk rigidity. PROM of all extremities is WFL. However, cogwheel rigidity is noted. AROM of the shoulders reveals a general 25%–30% loss in all motions. AROM at all other UE joints is WFL. AROM of LEs is WFL. However, movements are slower and require more effort as compared to the UE's.

The pt. presents with signs and symptoms consistent with the progression of Parkinson's disease. The patient would benefit from physical therapy to improve/maintain gait, maintenance of ADL abilities, maintenance/improvement of trunk ROM, and maintenance of extremity ROM.

The pt. would benefit from PT twice weekly for four to six weeks. Therapy sessions to include:

- ROM activities
- Transfer training
- Objective gait analysis/monitoring
- Gait training
- Home maintenance instruction

Organize, Relate, and Bracket

The initial task in the first step of the ORBIT model is to develop a problem list. In this particular case, the PTA might identify right foot drag, decreased arm swing, trunk and extremity rigidity, freezing, transfer and bed mobility impairment, and bradykinesia as the problems (**Figure 13.2**). Although the development of a problem list may seem to be stating the obvious, it does provide PTAs the opportunity to strip away details and focus on the clinical manifestations.

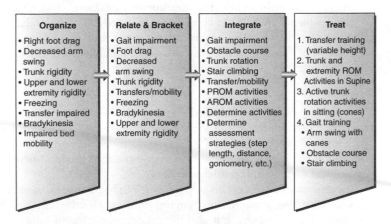

Organize	Relate & Bracket	Integrate	Treat

• Right foot drag
• Decreased arm swing
• Trunk rigidity
• Upper and lower extremity rigidity
• Freezing
• Transfer impaired
• Bradykinesia
• Impaired bed mobility
	• Gait impairment
	• Foot drag
	• Decreased arm swing
	• Trunk rigidity
	• Transfers/mobility
	• Freezing
	• Bradykinesia
	• Upper and lower extremity rigidity
		• Gait impairment
		• Obstacle course
		• Trunk rotation
		• Stair climbing
		• Transfer/mobility
		• PROM activities
		• AROM activities
		• Determine activities
		• Determine assessment strategies (step length, distance, goniometry, etc.)
			1. Transfer training (variable height)
			2. Trunk and extremity ROM Activities in Supine
			3. Active trunk rotation activities in sitting (cones)
			4. Gait training
			  • Arm swing with canes
			  • Obstacle course
			  • Stair climbing

Figure 13.2 ORBIT Example

The next task in this step—*relate and bracket*—enables the PTA to begin the important process of putting the patient's problem into clinical perspective. For instance, the plan of care calls for gait training. The PTA may relate the foot drag, decreased arm swing, and the trunk rigidity and bracket them with gait impairment. By doing so, the PTA may then be better able to develop therapeutic activities that address these issues in the broader context of gait rather than solely as individual problems. Similarly, the freezing, bradykinesia, and extremity rigidity might be related to each other and bracketed with the transfer and ROM issues.

Integrate

In the second step—*integrate*—the PTA begins the process of synthesizing the treatment session and activities. Because gait training was specified in the initial evaluation, the PTA begins to select the gait activities that might be most appropriate to address the previously identified and processed problems. In this case, the PTA may choose obstacle course activities that facilitate active hip and knee flexion, along with ankle dorsiflexion. Trunk rotation activities in standing and during gait, as well as stair climbing activities, may also be included.

This step also includes selecting appropriate assessment strategies. As stated earlier, PTAs must be able to discern the effects of their rehabilitation interventions. This occurs only through sound and objective assessment. In this case, objective assessment variables such as step length, gait distance, and goniometry were chosen.

Treat

The final step in the ORBIT model is to treat the patient. During this step, PTAs determine the sequence and types of interventions. For instance, in this case the PTA may decide to use stacking-cones activities to facilitate trunk rotation in sitting and start the treatment session with sit-to-stand transfer activities.

The important aspect of this step is that PTAs begin the treatment session with a plan in mind. This plan not only includes the type and sequence of interventions, but also the predetermination of important assessment strategies and techniques. By completing all steps of the ORBIT model, PTAs can better manage rehabilitation time, maximize rehabilitation potential, and maintain patient focus.

◀ Conclusion

The ORBIT model is one way that PTAs can organize themselves for the effective provision of physical therapy services. Indeed, other management models are available. However, the use of a formal management model is less important than the commitment to a systematic, well thought out approach to physical therapy care. Physical therapy is complex. Typically, several factors must be considered for even seemingly simple decisions.

The goal of this chapter—indeed of this entire text—is to illuminate the factors required to make clinical decisions and how best to apply various decision-making techniques. The physical therapy care delivery system is increasingly complex and is often fraught with opportunity for both success and failure. PTAs must always strive to provide effective care that reflects an understanding of their role in the healthcare system, demonstrates their level of training and education, and appreciates their important relationship with physical therapists.

The authors of this text have heard practicing PTAs give voice to the sentiment that clinically there is little difference between PTs and PTAs—that the biggest difference is that PTs can do evaluations and determine the plan of care, whereas PTAs cannot. Though this may seem true on the surface—and is often conveniently stated for administrative purposes—it is far from true. Clearly, the breadth and depth of physical therapists' education provides a foundation of support and direction for PTA provision of physical therapy care. Similarly, the level of physical therapist assistant education makes PTAs uniquely and singularly qualified to efficiently extend the therapeutic reach of physical therapists. By outlining the breadth of clinical decisions that must be made to provide effective physical therapy treatment, it should be clear that the PT–PTA relationship should always be open and continuously collaborative.

Index

A

active range of motion (AROM), 41,
 169, 172
 exercises, 19
age, 87, 96, 98, 106, 111, 113, 114, 115,
 142, 169
 pathology *vs.* old, 130
 related changes, 123, 124, 128
 related changes *vs.* medical
 condition, 129
Alzheimer's, 19, 131, 136
ambulation training, 29, 126, 132,
 143, 149
 assistive devices and, 33–34
 non-weight-bearing, 110
 progressive, 33–34
American Physical Therapy
 Association (APTA), 21
amputation, 142, 144, 145
 transtibial, 149–153
amyotrophic lateral sclerosis, 74
analog scales, 55
anatomy, 47, 83, 84, 86
 muscular, 89
anxiety, 33, 144
 recovery process and, 145
APTA. *See* American Physical Therapy
 Association
AROM. *See* active range of motion
arthritis, 88, 89, 100, 130
 osteo, 134

assessment, 13, 14, 146, 171, 174
 continuous, 6–7, 34, 46, 74
 key questions in gait, 35
 neurological disorders, tools,
 69–70
 of objective measures, 3, 6–7
 pediatric, tools, 113, 114
 psychological, 129
 of skin integrity, 143, 147
assistive devices, 29
 ambulation training and, 33–34
 effectiveness of, 34
 for gait training, 30, 31

B

balance, 30, 84, 89, 98, 109, 115, 127
 tests, 129
 training, 78, 83, 117
ball, 88
bed mobility, 19, 38, 40, 61, 78, 80, 81,
 131, 132, 137, 139, 143, 153, 156,
 165, 166
behavior
 modification, 111
 teaching, 143
bipolar technique, 58
Bircher, Wendy, 13
blindness, 19
blood pressure, 164
bradykinesia, 172, 174
Brunnstrom technique, 76, 77

C

cancer, 19, 110, 134, 165, 166
cardiac disease, 142
cardiopulmonary function, 83, 84, 89, 159
cardiorespiratory endurance, 124
case management, 169
    ORBIT, 170–171
CBC. *See* complete blood count
cells, 55
central biasing theory, 56, 57
central nervous system, impairment, 17
cerebral palsy, 107
    athetoid/spastic, 117
cerebrovascular accident (CVA), 4, 29, 65, 68, 73, 78, 130, 131, 134, 143, 170
children, 145
    with disabilities, 109, 111
    schools for, with disabilities, 107, 108, 110, 111
    social concerns and, 111
cholecystectomy, 159
clinical decision-making, 7, 42–43, 169, 175
    cognitive ability and, 131
    critical care patient and, 156–157
    critical care patient and, limits, 164
    electrical stimulation and, 8, 57, 59
    electrical stimulation and, limits, 59
    ethical conflict and, 25
    factors, 3
    in gait training, 35
    gait training and, limits, 37
    geriatric physical therapy and, 127
    geriatric physical therapy and, limits, 132–133
    isokinetic exercise and, 94
    isometric exercise and, 94
    isotonic exercise, 92
    neurological disorders and, 65, 66, 71, 73
    neurological disorders and, limits, 76–77
    objective measures and, 69
    orthotic training and, limits, 148
    pediatric physical therapy and, 108–109, 115
    pediatric physical therapy and, limits, 116
    prosthetic training and, limits, 148
    prosthetic/orthotic training and, 147, 148
    SOAP and, 13, 14
    task analysis and, 74, 75
    therapeutic exercise and, 85, 86, 88, 89, 90, 92, 95–96
    therapeutic exercise and, limits, 98–99
    thermotherapy and, limits, 48
cognitive ability, 128
    clinical decision-making and, 131
cognitive development, 1, 115
cold pack, 44
comfort, 9
    level, 127
    patient, 59
    zone, 111
communication, 69, 137
    customizing, 17
    factors precipitating, 15
    interdisciplinary, 4, 108–109, 111
    nonverbal, 17
    with parents, 112
    with patient, 16–18, 19
    with PT, 11, 12, 15, 16, 37, 99, 109–110, 112, 115, 116, 146, 147, 148, 156
    strategies, 17, 18
    style, 18
community programs, 128
complete blood count (CBC)
    changes in, 159
    values, 160–161

complications, preventing, 131
congestive heart failure, 130
coordination, 30, 83, 98
coping mechanism, of parents, 112
coronary bypass surgery, 19, 87
critical care, 155
critical care patient
    clinical decision-making and, 156–157
    limits on clinical decisions and, 164
    medical devices/equipment and,
        155, 157, 158
    objective measures and, 159–164
    physical therapy and, 155–156
    physical therapy evaluation and,
        166–168
    recovery process and, 156
    rehabilitation environment and,
        157–158
    treatment goals and, 156, 157
cryotherapy, 16, 41, 44
cuff weights, 86, 95
CVA. *See* cerebrovascular accident
cyanosis, 159, 162

D

Daily Adjustable Progressive Resistive
    Exercise (DAPRE), 93
daily living, activities of, 4, 5, 6, 66, 87
DAPRE. *See* Daily Adjustable
    Progressive Resistive Exercise
Delorme technique, 93
dementia, 131
depression, 132, 144
development
    cognitive, 1, 115
    delay of, 119
    neurological, 76, 77, 107, 113, 171
    understanding normal, 115
diabetes, 142
diagnosis, 3, 30, 87, 107, 142
diaphoresis, 162

digital camera, 55
digitizers, portable, 55
disabilities
    accepting, 145
    children with, 109, 111
    schools for children with, 107, 108,
        110, 111
documentation, 88, 129; *See also*
    progress notes
    inappropriate, 23
    and interdisciplinary team, 13
dumbbells, 86
dynametrics, 55
dynamometer speed, 94

E

ECG. *See* electrocardiogram
edema, 16, 58, 93, 130, 146, 148
    control, 54
education, 17, 113
    continuing, 7
    patient, 143, 145, 148, 149, 165
    PTA, 7, 42, 76, 107
efficiency, 169
electrical stimulation
    clinical decisions and, 8, 57, 59
    equipment, 54
    knowledge/expertise and, 55–56,
        58, 59
    limits on clinical decisions and, 59
    muscle contraction and, 58, 59
    muscle contraction and,
        parameters, 58
    objective measures and, 55
    pain management and, 56–57
    pain management theories and, 56
    parameters of, 53, 56
    patient needs and, 55
    physical therapy evaluation and, 60–63
    rehabilitation environment and, 54
    treatment goals of, 54

electrocardiogram (ECG), 158
electrode
  pain management and, placement, 57
  placement, 53, 59
empathy, 145
endogenous opiate theory, 56
endurance, 83, 84, 89, 117, 156
  cardiorespiratory, 124
equilibrium, 115, 125
equipment
  critical care patient and, 155, 157, 158
  electrical stimulation, 54
  geriatric physical therapy, 127
  neurological disorders and, 67–68
  pediatric physical therapy, 108
  therapeutic exercise, 86
erythema, 16
ethical behavior, 21, 23, 26–27
  continuum view of, 22
  private practice and, 24
ethical conflict, 23, 24
  clinical decision-making process and, 25
evaluation
  critical care patient physical therapy, 166–168
  electrical stimulation physical therapy, 60–63
  gait, 71, 115
  gait training physical therapy, 38–40
  geriatric physical therapy, 134–139
  initial, 169, 170
  neurological disorders physical therapy, 78–82
  Parkinson's disease physical therapy, 172–173
  pediatric physical therapy, 118–121
  prosthetic training physical therapy, 149–153
  therapeutic exercise, process, 84–85

therapeutic exercise physical therapy, 101–104
thermotherapy physical therapy, 49–52
exercise(s), 18, 100; *See also* therapeutic exercise
  AROM, 19
  concepts, 89
  Frenkel's, 76
  home, programs, 6
  impact of, 96
  intensity of, 142
  muscle-setting, 93
  open chain/closed chain, 91, 96, 147
  programs, 87
  resistive, 12, 16, 98
  resistive, dosage, 93
eyesight, 125

F
fainting, 168
fall prevention, 125, 129
FAMS. *See* Functional Assessment of Multiple Sclerosis
fatigue, 87, 96, 110, 159
finance, 23
fitness, 87, 96
flexibility, 83
Frenkel's exercises, 76
frequency, 53, 58, 89
fun, pediatric physical therapy and, 110, 111, 115, 116
Functional Assessment of Multiple Sclerosis (FAMS), 70

G
gait, 156, 172, 173
  assessment, 35
  deviations/compensations, 36, 148
  evaluation, 71, 115
gait training, 3, 4, 9, 18, 68, 114, 124, 141, 174
  assistive devices for, 30, 31

clinical decision-making in, 35
knowledge/expertise and, 34–36
limits on clinical decisions and, 37
objective measures and, 32
objective progress in, 71, 72
objective spatial parameters and, 32
patient needs and, 31
physical therapy evaluation and, 38–40
rehabilitation environment and, 30–31
symmetry and, 33
treatment goals of, 29, 30
gate control theory, 56, 57
geriatric patient
age-related changes in, 124
home care for, 126
medical history and, 130
needs, 127–128
psychological issues of, 123, 127, 128, 129, 132
social concerns of, 127, 128, 129
treatment plans for, 132
geriatric physical therapy, 123
clinical decision-making and, 127
equipment, 127
evaluation, 134–139
knowledge/expertise and, 129–132
limits on clinical decisions and, 132–133
objective measures and, 128–129
patient needs and, 125, 127–128
prescription and, 132
rehabilitation environment and, 125–127
treatment goals and, 124–125
goniometry, 88, 128, 146, 174

H
healing, 42
soft tissue, 54
hearing loss, 17, 119

hemiparesis, 138
hemiplegia, 118
hemoglobin, 159
hip, 134
flexion, 149
fracture, 130, 136
replacement, 19
home care
for geriatric patient, 126
for pediatric patient, 107, 109
hospitals, 5, 23
acute care, 107, 110, 117, 125, 159
inpatient rehabilitation, 108
hot packs, 41, 46, 49
usage patterns of, 43–44
hypotonicity, upper extremity, 76

I
ice pack, 44
IEP. *See* Individual Educational Program
imagination, 67, 96, 106, 116
immaturity, emotional, 110
independence, 143
levels of, 33
loss of, 128, 132
Individual Educational Program (IEP), 113
Individual Family Support Plan, 113
inexperience, 33
infarctions, myocardial, 128
infection, 130, 136
inflammation, 16, 42, 44
infrared, 45, 46
instruction
inability to understand, 110
patient needs, 18
integration, 171, 174
integrity, 23, 25
assessment of skin, 143, 147

interdisciplinary team
    communication with, 4, 108–109, 111
    written documentation and, 13
intervention, 3, 4, 13, 66; *See also*
        treatment; treatment goals
    alternate/blended, strategies, 76
    customized, 68, 71, 72
    prioritizing, 156, 171
    selection, 74
    strategies, 77, 107, 110
intracranial pressure (ICP), 158
intravenous lines (IV), 157, 167
iontophoresis, 9, 59
isokinetic exercise, 90, 91, 93
    clinical decision-making and, 94
isokinetic strengthening, 9, 89
isometric exercise, 90, 91, 93
    clinical decision-making and, 94
isotonic exercise, 90, 91, 94
    clinical decision-making and, 92
    dosage, 93
IV. *See* intravenous lines

J
joint, 44, 84, 130
    motion, 94
    ROM, 4, 156

K
Kettenbach, Ginge, 13
kinesiology, 83, 85, 86, 89
knee, 100
    sprain, 103
    total, arthroplasty, 38
knowledge
    clinical, 3, 7–8
    electrical stimulation and clinical,
        55–56, 58, 59
    gait training and clinical, 34–36
    geriatric physical therapy and
        clinical, 129–132

neurological disorders and clinical,
    71, 73–74
new, 15
orthotic training and clinical, 147–148
pediatric physical therapy and
    clinical, 114–116
prosthetic training and clinical,
    147–148
therapeutic exercise and clinical, 89,
    90, 91, 95, 96, 98
thermotherapy and clinical, 46–48

L
language, difference, 17
learning
    lifelong, 15
    peer, 7
    styles, 18
legislation, 21, 24
leukemia, 117
life, 15
    expectancy, 123
    quality of, 125
    stage, 88
    style, 88, 124, 143
limb
    phantom, pain, 144
    residual, 145
    shaping of residual, 141, 143, 148
locomotion, human, 29
longevity, 123, 125
loss, 144
    hearing, 17, 119
    of spouse/independence, 128, 132

M
manifestation list
    patient problem/clinical, 170, 173
    prioritizing, 171
manual muscle testing (MMT), 88, 90,
    91–92, 128, 146

medical condition, 125–126, 156
  age-related changes *vs.*, 129
  pediatric physical therapy and,
    108, 110
  secondary, 127, 128
medical devices, 167
  critical care patient and, 155, 157, 158
medical history, 88, 96, 98, 128, 137, 142
  geriatric patient and, 130
meningitis, 165
meniscectomy, 100
mental status, 30, 96, 111, 129, 169
Minimum Record of Disability
    (MRD), 69
MMT. *See* manual muscle testing
monopolar technique, 58
mood, 93
motivation, 128, 132, 144
motor
  control, 107, 113
  impairment, 143
MRD. *See* Minimum Record of
    Disability
MS. *See* multiple sclerosis
MSFC. *See* Multiple Sclerosis Function
    Composite
MSIS-29. *See* Multiple Sclerosis
    Impact Scale
MSQLI. *See* Multiple Sclerosis Quality
    of Life Inventory
multiple sclerosis (MS), 65, 69–70
Multiple Sclerosis Function Composite
    (MSFC), 70
Multiple Sclerosis Impact Scale
    (MSIS-29), 70
Multiple Sclerosis Quality of Life
    Inventory (MSQLI), 70
muscle(s), 29, 34, 76, 77, 97, 98
  anatomy of, 89
  atrophy, 131
  control, 70

electric stimulation and,
    contraction, 58, 59
electric stimulation parameters and,
    contraction, 58
manual, testing, 88, 90, 91–92,
    128, 146
mass, 124
resistance arm and, load, 95
setting exercise, 93
soreness, 87, 96
strength, 4, 54, 89, 91, 106, 156
tone, 107, 113, 115, 139
musculoskeletal factors, 29, 34
myocardial infarction, 130

N

nasogastric (NG) tube, 157
NDT. *See* neurodevelopmental
    techniques
neurodevelopmental techniques
    (NDT), 76, 77, 107, 171
neurological development, 76, 77,
    107, 113
neurological disorders
  assessment tools, 69–70
  clinical decision-making and, 65,
    66, 71, 73
  equipment and, 67–68
  knowledge/expertise and, 71, 73–74
  limits on clinical decisions and,
    76–77
  objective measures and, 69, 70, 71
  patient needs and, 68–69
  in pediatric patient, 107, 114–115
  physical therapy evaluation and,
    78–82
  progressive/nonprogressive, 73–74
  rehabilitation environment and,
    67–68
  sequelae and, 65, 66, 68, 107
  treatment goals and, 65–66, 67, 77

neuromuscular factors, 29, 34
NG. *See* nasogastric tube
nursing homes, 5, 23

O

obesity, 45
objective measures, 13
    clinical decision-making and, 69
    critical care patient and, 159–164
    electrical stimulation and, 55
    gait training and, 32
    geriatric physical therapy and,
        128–129
    neurological disorders and, 69, 70, 71
    pediatric physical therapy and,
        112–114
    physical therapy and, 69
    prosthetic/orthotic training and,
        146–147
    therapeutic exercise and, 88–89
    thermotherapy and, 45–46
    utilization/assessment of, 3, 6–7
observation, 29, 88
ORBIT
    application, 171–175
    case management, 170–171
    example, 173
orthopedic condition, 106, 125
orthostatic hypotension, 164
orthotic devices, 141
    choosing of, 146
    donning/doffing, 142, 143
    fitting, 148
    sequelae and, 147
    treatment goals and, 141–143
orthotic training, 141
    clinical decision-making and, 147, 148
    on clinical decisions and, 148
    knowledge/expertise and, 147–148
    limits on clinical decisions and, 148
    monitoring, 147

    objective measures and, 146–147
    patient needs and, 144–145
    psychological issues and, 144–145
    rehabilitation environment and,
        143–144
osteoarthritis, 100
Oxford technique, 93
oxygenation, 159

P

pain, 93, 110, 146
    phantom limb, 144
    questionnaires, 55
    relief, 54
    shoulder, 101
pain management, 12, 19, 30, 42, 106
    electrical stimulation and, 55–57
    electrode placement and, 57
    theories and electrical
        stimulation, 56
parallel bars, 34
parameters
    of electrical stimulation, 53, 56
    gait training, 32
    muscle contraction and electrical
        stimulation, 58
    objective, 29
    treatment, 3, 13
parents
    communication with, 112
    coping mechanism of, 112
    involvement of, 111–112
Parkinson's disease, 171
    physical therapy evaluation, 172–173
pathology, 83, 90, 96, 113
    aging *vs.*, 130
    function and, 114
patient, 6; *See also* critical care patient;
    geriatric patient; pediatric patient
    altered, status, 16
    comfort, 59

communication with, 16–18, 19
education, 143, 145, 148, 149, 165
effort of, 5–6
problem/clinical manifestation list,
170, 173
response, 87
therapeutic exercise and, 87–88
thermotherapy and, 44–45
patient needs, 3, 30, 169–170
analyzing, 2, 3
electrical stimulation and, 55
gait training and, 31
geriatric physical therapy and, 125,
127–128
instruction, 18
neurological disorders and, 68–69
orthotic training and, 144–145
prosthetic training and, 144–145
PDAs. *See* personal digital assistants
pediatric patient
assessment tools for, 113, 114
common problems of, 106
home care for, 107, 109
needs of, 110–112
neurological disorders in, 107,
114–115
rehabilitation environment and,
107–110
therapeutic exercise for, 106
treatment plan for, 107
pediatric physical therapy, 105
clinical decision-making and,
108–109, 115
equipment for, 108
evaluation, 118–121
fun/entertainment and, 110, 111,
115, 116
knowledge/expertise and, 114–116
limits on clinical decisions and, 116
medical condition and, 108, 110
objective measures and, 112–114

treatment goals of, 106–107,
115, 116
peripheral vascular disease
(PVD), 142
personal digital assistants
(PDAs), 13
personal goals, 125
personnel
ancillary, 23
inappropriately trained, 24
pharmacology, 156
physical therapist (PT), 7, 9, 58, 59,
69, 90
communication with, 11, 12, 15, 16,
37, 99, 109–110, 112, 115, 116,
146, 147, 148, 156
pediatric specialist, 105, 109
PTA and, 175
physical therapy, 1; *See also* geriatric
physical therapy; pediatric
physical therapy
complexity of, 23
critical care patient and, 155–156
critical care patient and, evaluation,
166–168
electrical stimulation and, evaluation, 60–63
gait training and, evaluation, 38–40
neurological disorders and,
evaluation, 78–82
objective measures and, 69
Parkinson's disease, evaluation,
172–173
prescriptive, 9, 42, 48, 105
prosthetic training and, evaluation,
149–153
refusal of, 23
therapeutic exercise and, evaluation,
101–104
thermotherapy and, evaluation,
49–52

physical therapy assistant (PTA),
  21, 22, 26
  becoming, 1–2
  education, 7, 42, 76, 107
  PT and, 175
  supervision, 23, 24
physical therapy technician, 1, 7
plyometrics, 96–97
pneumonia, 165
PNF. *See* proprioceptive neuromuscular facilitation
posture, 6, 94, 107
  reflex and, 114
PRE. *See* progressive resistive exercise
premorbid condition, 6, 87
preprosthetic training, 141–142
prescription, 169
  geriatric physical therapy and, 132
  physical therapy and, 9, 42, 48, 105
  of therapeutic exercise, 83–84
prevention, 18
  contracture, 141, 143, 148
private practice, 5, 23
  ethics in, 24
prognosis, understanding, 114
progress notes, 12–13, 33, 69, 129;
  See also documentation
progressive ambulation training,
  33–34
progressive resistive exercise (PRE),
  98
PROM activities, 41, 156, 172
proprioception, 97, 113
proprioceptive neuromuscular
  facilitation (PNF), 76, 77, 96
  benefits of, 97
  treatment considerations for, 98
prosthetic devices
  choosing of, 146
  donning/doffing, 142, 143
  fitting, 148

  sequelae and, 147
  treatment goals and, 141–143
prosthetic training, 141
  clinical decision-making and,
    147, 148
  knowledge/expertise and, 147–148
  limits on clinical decisions and, 148
  monitoring devices for, 146
  objective measures and, 146–147
  patient needs and, 144–145
  physical therapy evaluation and,
    149–153
  psychological issues and, 144–145
  rehabilitation environment and,
    143–144
psychology, 29, 34, 129
  geriatric patient and, 123, 127, 128,
    129, 132
  prosthetic/orthotic training and,
    144–145
psychosocial stressors, 123, 129, 132
PTA. *See* physical therapist; physical
  therapy assistant
pulmonary status, 156, 162
pulse duration, 58, 59
PVD. *See* peripheral vascular disease

R
ramp time, 58
range of motion (ROM), 4, 30, 47, 83,
  90, 106, 117, 141, 142, 146, 173;
  See also active range of motion
  joint, 4, 156
RBC. *See* red blood cells
recovery process, 90, 142, 143, 144
  anxiety and, 145
  critical care patient and, 156
red blood cells (RBC), 159
reflex, 113
  tonic vibratory, 76
  tonic/postural, 115

regulatory agency, 23
rehabilitation
   centers, 5, 23, 107
   critical care patient and, environ-
      ment, 157–158
   electrical stimulation and, environ-
      ment, 54
   environment, 3, 4–5, 14
   gait training and, environment, 30–31
   geriatric physical therapy and,
      environment, 125–127
   inpatient, hospitals, 108
   neurological disorders and,
      environment, 67–68
   orthotic training and, environment,
      143–144
   pediatric patient and, environment,
      107–110
   process, 143, 144, 146, 148
   prosthetic training and,
      environment, 143–144
   therapeutic exercise and,
      environment, 85–87
   thermotherapy and, environment,
      43–44
relaxation, 42
renal disease, 142
resistance, 12, 16
   exercise, 12, 16, 98
   exercise dosage, 93
   muscle load and, arm, 95
resources, 4, 5, 67
respiratory problems, 45, 159
   signs of, 162
respiratory rate, 162
response
   patient, 87
   to therapy, 16
retirement, 128
rigidity, 172, 174
role-playing, 21

ROM. *See* range of motion
Rood technique, 76, 77
rulers, flexible, 55

S
safety, 9, 11, 30, 33, 86, 124, 143
schools, 5
   for children with disabilities, 107,
      108, 110, 111
   public, 109
seizure, 119
self-management, strategies, 66
sensation, 70
sensory perception, 113
sepsis, postsurgical, 159
sequelae
   cascading effects of, 66, 67
   decision-making query on, and
      function relationship, 75
   function and, 74
   neurological disorders and, 65, 66,
      68, 107
   prosthetic/orthotic devices and, 147
serum electrolyte level, 156
   changes in, 159
   values, 161
Shamus, Eric, 13
shoulder, 169
   adhesive capsulitis of, 4, 41, 42, 49
   complex disorder, 90
   pain, 101
shrinker garments, 143, 145
Sinemet, 172
skills, 107
   maintaining/ updating, 7
skin care, 143, 147
SOAP. *See* Subjective/Objective/
     Assessment/Plan
social concerns
   children and, 111
   of geriatric patient, 127, 128, 129

soft tissue
  extensibility, 42
  healing, 54
spasm, management, 42
specialty clinics, 5
speech therapy, 14
Standards for Ethical Conduct for the
    Physical Therapist Assistant, 21,
    22, 26
state regulations, supervision and, 109
Stern, Debra, 13
strength(s), 2, 115, 117, 141, 146
  isokinetic, activity, 9, 98
  monitoring, gain, 55
  muscle, 4, 54, 89, 91, 106, 156
  therapeutic exercise and, 90
  training, 83
stress, 23
stretching, 42, 90, 115, 157
stroke, 131
Subjective/Objective/Assessment/
    Plan (SOAP), 168
  clinical decision-making and, 13, 14
supervision, 69
  PTA, 23, 24
  state regulations and, 109
supportive services, 112

T
task analysis, clinical decision-making
    and, 74, 75
TBI. *See* traumatic brain injury
teaching strategies, 127
technology, 14
tendonitis, 49
TENS. *See* transcutaneous electrical
    nerve stimulation
tests
  balance, 129
  manual muscle, 88, 90, 91–92,
    128, 146

theory(ies)
  central biasing, 56
  electrical stimulation and pain
    management, 56
  endogenous opiate, 56
  gate control, 56, 57
therapeutic exercise, 3, 139; *See also*
    exercise(s)
  body position/weight placement
    and, 95
  choice of, 87–88
  clinical decision-making and, 85, 86,
    88, 89, 90, 92, 95–96
  components of, 83
  equipment, 86
  evaluation process and, 84–85
  function and, 87
  intensity/duration/frequency
    and, 89
  isometric/isotonic/isokinetic, 90,
    91, 93, 94
  knowledge/expertise and, 89, 90, 91,
    95, 96, 98
  limits on clinical decisions and,
    98–99
  objective measures and, 88–89
  patient needs and, 87–88
  for pediatric patient, 106
  physical therapy evaluation and,
    101–104
  prescription and, 83–84
  rehabilitation environment and,
    85–87
  strengthening, 90
  treatment goals of, 84, 85, 88
therapeutic ions, transcutaneous
    delivery of, 54
therapy; *See also specific therapies*
  modalities of, 16
  response to, 16
  speech, 14

thermotherapy
  contraindications/precautions
    for, 45
  depth of penetration of, modalities,
    46, 47
  knowledge/expertise and, 46–48
  limits on clinical decisions and, 48
  modalities of, 43
  objective measures and, 45–46
  patient needs and, 44–45
  physical therapy evaluation and, 49–52
  rehabilitation environment and, 43–44
  time/positioning decisions and, 47
  treatment goals of, 41, 42, 45–47
third party payers, 13, 23, 66
time management, 13, 47
TKA. *See* total knee arthroplasty
total knee arthroplasty (TKA), 38
toys, 108
transcutaneous electrical nerve stimu-
    lation (TENS), 54, 55
traumatic brain injury (TBI), 65, 78,
    87, 118, 119, 143, 167
treatment, 3, 13, 171, 174–175; *See
    also* intervention
  considerations for PNF, 98
  effectiveness of, 87
  philosophies, 76, 77
  routine, 15
  schools of thought, 76
treatment goals, 4, 15
  achieving, 112
  critical care patient and, 156, 157
  of electrical stimulation, 54
  of gait training, 29, 30
  geriatric physical therapy and,
    124–125
  neurological disorders and, 65–66,
    67, 77
  orthotic devices and, 141–143
  of pediatric physical therapy,
    106–107, 115, 116
  prioritizing, 66, 85
  prosthetic devices and, 141–143
  of therapeutic exercise, 84, 85, 88
  of thermotherapy, 41, 42, 45–46
treatment plan(s), 3, 37, 42, 65, 77, 98,
    171, 174
  alteration of, 16
  customized, 169
  for geriatric patient, 132
  for pediatric patient, 107
tremor, 172

U
ultrasound, 5, 41, 46, 47, 49

V
vital signs, 114, 128, 131, 156, 167
  changes in, 159
  normal values of, 163, 164
voltage, 54

W
walker, 33, 34
waveform, 53
weight(s)
  bearing status, 30, 37, 38
  cuff, 86, 95
  non, bearing ambulation
    training, 110
  therapeutic exercise and,
    placement, 95
Whipple procedure, 166
wound, 55
  management, 141
wrapping techniques, 143, 145